R
'26.8
'16
197

Hospice and Palliative Care

Questions and Answers

Virginia F. Sendor and Patrice M. O'Connor

The Scarecrow Press, Inc.
Lanham, Md., & London
1997

SCARECROW PRESS, INC.

Published in the United States of America
by Scarecrow Press, Inc.
4720 Boston Way
Lanham, Maryland 20706

DISCLAIMER: This book is intended as a reference work only. It is not
intended as a substitute for medical or legal advice.

British Library Cataloguing in Publication Information Available

Library of Congress Cataloging-in-Publication Data

Sendor, Virginia F.
  Hospice and palliative care : questions and answers / Virginia F. Sendor and
Patrice M. O'Connor.
    p. cm.
  Includes bibliographical references and index.
  ISBN 0-8108-3308-5 (alk. paper)
  1. Hospice care. 2. Hospices (Terminal care). 3. Terminal care. I.
O'Connor, Patrice M. II. Title.
R726.8.S46 1997   97-10620
362.1'756—dc21   CIP

ISBN 0-8108-3308-5 (pbk.: alk. paper)

We dedicate this book
to
The Patients and Their Families
Past,
Present,
and Future...

The authors wish to express appreciation for the support and encouragement of The American Institute of Life-Threatening Illness and Loss, a division of The Foundation of Thanatology, in the preparation of this volume. Thanatology, a new subspecialty of medicine, is involved in scientific and humanistic inquiries and the application of the knowledge derived therefrom to the subjects of the psychological aspects of dying; reactions to loss, death, and grief; and recovery from bereavement.

The Foundation of Thanatology is dedicated to advancing the cause of enlightened health care for the terminally ill patient and his family. The Foundation's orientation is a positive one based on the philosophy of fostering a more mature acceptance and understanding of death and the problems of grief and the more effective and humane management and treatment of the dying patient and his bereaved family members.

CONTENTS

What is meant by "quality assurance" in the Hospice program?

Disposal of controlled drugs: What happens to the unused medication(s) in the home when the physician changes the prescription or the patient dies?

How will the spiritual needs of patients, families, and significant others be met by the Hospice program? How does Hospice handle the spiritual needs of an atheist or a metaphysician?

What is "unfinished business"?

What is a patient and family bill of rights?

What is meant by "Informed Consent"? How is this documented?

What happens to the rights of minor patients? What happens to the rights of the incompetent patient?

What are the benefits of Hospice services for the family?

Will the Hospice permit the family to participate in caring for the patient?

Can Hospice assist the patient and family before the patient is medically ready to be admitted to the Hospice program?

Why is having a primary caregiver so important to the patient in a Hospice program?

Will the Hospice be available to the patient and family whenever they need Hospice services?

How can Hospice help family/caregiver(s) who are stressed out and cannot cope?

What are the needs of the terminally ill patient and family for intimacy and sexuality?

What are some of the things a patient and family might do to maximize the time that is left?

Under what circumstances is a Hospice patient transferred from the home to inpatient care in a hospital (or in a nursing home)?

What are some other issues of concern for people with AIDS in regard to Hospice care?

What do Hospices do to educate and train their staff (including volunteers and contract staff) who work with HIV/AIDS patients?

Is the Hospice philosophy and care appropriate for people with AIDS, their families, and significant others? How can Hospice services help them?

Do most Hospices accept persons with AIDS into their programs? Are the Hospice admission criteria different for persons with various terminal conditions including HIV/AIDS?

What can a Hospice program offer persons with AIDS, their families, and significant others? What is "migration home" syndrome?

Is Hospice care different for people with HIV/AIDS than for people with cancer or other terminal conditions?

What are the bereavement implications of the "multiple losses" experienced by people living with HIV/AIDS, their families, and significant others?

How has the profile of persons living with AIDS changed over the past ten years?

What are AIDS Service Organizations (ASOs)? Can Hospices and ASOs collaborate to benefit the HIV/AIDS population?

Can you suggest some informative reading material about HIV/AIDS?

Who can be referred to a Hospice program? Who can make these referrals?

If the patient or family is not sure the patient is ready for Hospice care, can they call the Hospice for information?

What needs to be in place before the patient/family is admitted to the Hospice?

What do the patient and family promise to provide the Hospice program before admission?

What does the physician have to offer the terminally ill patient and family? What is "Palliative Care"?

How can the physician facilitate the patient's and family's well-being through Hospice care?

What are the advantages and disadvantages of Hospice care for the terminally ill patient and family?

Will the patient have to change doctors? What is the relationship of the patient's attending physician and the Hospice physician? What is the role of the attending physician when the patient is in the Hospice program? Do Hospice physicians really make house calls? What are some of the factors that influence the attending physician to relinquish care when the patient is admitted to the Hospice program?

How does the patient's attending physician feel about giving a six-month prognosis for the Medicare certified Hospice program? How does the attending physician feel about referring a patient to Hospice? Why do some physicians wait until the death of the patient is imminent before referring the patient to Hospice?

Does Hospice force religion or spirituality on its patients?

What is the importance of symptom relief in terminal care?

How can the physical pain of a terminally ill patient be adequately alleviated?

Will I become addicted to narcotics if I take them for pain? Will they hasten the end? Does Hospice use too much morphine?

How does the Hospice physician feel about honoring patient and family requests concerning "patient self-determination": the health care proxy, do-not-resuscitate orders, living wills, and the durable power of attorney?

What happens at the time of the patient's death in a Hospice program?

Is there a state Hospice organization in my state?
Are there other agencies that might be able to help me?
Can you suggest some books for me to read?

ACKNOWLEDGMENTS

We are indeed indebted to the following individuals and groups for helping us truly learn what Hospice is all about. Our deepest thanks to:

The patients, their families, and significant others who were part of the St. Luke's Palliative Care Program and the Long Island Foundation for Hospice Care and Research, who were so gracious in permitting us to walk with them during a precious time of their lives. The staff and volunteers of Hospice and Palliative Care teams, who taught us what caring is all about. Our family and friends, who listened to all our tales and gave us the strength to continue in this field.

Dame Cicely Saunders, M.D., who taught us that compassionate care for the terminally ill is possible in modern medicine. Dr. Austin H. Kutscher, who gave us the opportunity to explore, express, and share the full meaning of Hospice and Palliative Care. Dr. Wendy W. Brown and Dr. Michael E. Frederich, for their professional response and the sharing of their expertise by responding to the questions in "Physicians Address Issues of Palliative Care."

Jane Weber and Paul R. Brenner, for sharing their professionalism and experiences with AIDS and Alzheimer's Disease in the Hospice program. The Rev. Stanert L. Dransfield, for sharing his thoughts on bereavement in the Hospice program. Dr. Elisabeth Kübler-Ross, for her patience and inspiration as teacher and mentor. Rosemary J. Hürzeler and the Rev. John W. Abbott, who helped point the way during my introduction to Hospice. Paul R. Brenner, who also shared with me and provided support in the process of developing a Hospice program, and later. Burke W. Deadrich, who made me aware of the nuances of Hospice and development. Philip G. DiSorbo, whose expertise was invaluable during the intricate licensing and Medicare Certification process, and beyond. Jules

Bernstein, Dolores Engelhardt, and Oliver Schepers, who taught and guided me through the political process. Arthur J. Kremer, Esq., and Jill Rosen-Nikoloff, Esq., for providing guidance and sharing their legal expertise.

The Rev. Carleton Sweetser, for his innovative approach to Hospice by introducing the scattered-bed model of Hospice care, and for his support, over the years, of both the program and staff. The Dominican Sisters of Sparkill, who taught me the true meaning of total patient care. The International Work Group in Death, Dying, and Bereavement, who continue to support and challenge.

John P. Breen, J. Kevin Meneilly, Esq., and the support staff of Massapequa General Hospital, for "being there" for me in so many ways and for sharing their professional expertise. Rabbi Melvin Keiffer and Rabbi Barry Dov Lerner, for their ongoing inspiration, encouragement, and support along the uphill road. John Bernstein, Mary Smith, and Thelma Weinberg, for creative networking and helping us meet our deadlines. My husband, Bernard T. Sendor, who has encouraged and supported me in following my dreams.

Truly, Hospice Palliative Care is all about networking, caring, and sharing. We cannot do it alone.

Virginia F. Sendor, MS, MPA
President
Long Island Foundation for Hospice Care and Research, Inc.

Patrice M. O'Connor, RN, MA, CNA
Palliative Care Consultant
St. Luke's/Roosevelt Hospital Center

PREFACE

Few of us are strangers to terminal illness. We are living in a time when almost everyone has lost a loved one or friend to cancer, Alzheimer's Disease, AIDS, or some other terminal illness.

Feelings of anguish and helplessness often are overwhelming as we struggle to care for our terminally ill loved one and then attempt to deal with our own grief and sense of loss.

Easing pain and compassionately ministering to the needs of the terminally ill, their families, and significant others is the purpose of the Hospice program. Hospice is not a place; it is a philosophy. It is a special kind of caring when cure is no longer possible—involving people who are responsive and sensitive to the unique needs of terminally ill patients, their families, and significant others.

Hospice emphasizes the most comfortable, natural environment for those confronted with a terminal disease. Wherever the Hospice care is provided—at home, in a hospital, a nursing home, or elsewhere—the philosophy of Hospice is consistent: to ease pain, manage the symptoms of the terminal illness and related conditions, and provide comfort to enhance the quality of life—not only for those facing death but also for their families and significant others. The emphasis is not just on physical pain but "total pain"—which can be mental, physical, spiritual, social, legal, or financial.

A patient and family confronted with a medical diagnosis of serious illness and a condition that may be terminal, go through a time of deep distress and anguish, confusion and despair. Frequently, there is an initial shock, numbness, and disbelief. Then the questions start to come:

- What do I do?
- Where can I get the information I need?
- Whom shall I talk to?

- What is a Hospice?
- How can I find a Hospice program near me?
- How can I get into a Hospice program?
- What kind of care will I get?
- What is the difference between care in the Hospice program and the care I would get in a hospital or nursing home?
- Who provides the care?
- How much does it cost?
- Who pays for this?

. . . and the questions continue to come.

This book presents the answers to actual questions asked by concerned and exhausted patients, their families, and significant others in crisis who are having difficulty coping with death and dying, which really is about life and living.

The answers to these questions evolved from our personal and professional observations and hands-on experiences. Technical information has been resourced from actual Hospice operations manuals and other pertinent literature. Resources include the American Academy of Hospice and Palliative Medicine; Capital District Hospice, Inc.; the National Hospice Organization, Inc.; the New York State Hospice Association, Inc.; Choice in Dying, Inc.; Children's Hospice International, Inc.; the Hospice Association of America; the St. Luke's/Roosevelt Hospital Center Palliative Care Program; the Long Island Foundation for Hospice Care and Research, Inc., and others.

We sincerely hope this book will help answer your questions and define and clarify any misconceptions about what Hospice care *is* and *is not*.

We hope we have presented the case that Hospice care *is* a legitimate, viable alternative to conventional curative care for the terminally ill, their families, and significant others. Even so, we are the first to admit that a Hospice program may not be appropriate for all patients medically diagnosed with a terminal illness. Hospice is not a panacea; it is not an end-all and be-all for all people at all times. Even for the same "patient/family unit," Hospice care that might not be appropriate at a particular time might be best for them at another time.

In the words of Dame Cicely Saunders, M.D., the founder and medical director of St. Christopher's Hospice in Sydenham, near London, England:

> You matter because you are you. You matter to the last moment of your life, and we will do all we can, not only to help you die peacefully, but also to live until you die.

1
WHAT IS HOSPICE?

A. INTRODUCTION

1. What is Hospice? What are the goals of Hospice?
2. What is the history of Hospice? How did it start?

Q: What is Hospice? What are the goals of Hospice?

Hospice is not a place or a building. It is a philosophy, a special kind of caring when cure is no longer possible.

Hospice is a coordinated interdisciplinary program of life-affirming compassionate care and supportive services for terminally ill individuals, their families, and significant others.

Hospice considers the ill person and the family as a whole. The patient and family are considered to be the "unit of care." Hospice addresses the physical, emotional, spiritual, and social—as well as economic and practical—needs of patients, their families, and significant others.

Hospice services are intended for persons with a limited life expectancy who are medically diagnosed as having a terminal illness. To be admitted into a Medicare certified Hospice program, the prognosis must be six months or less to live.

Hospice offers care to people of all ages, to children as well as adults, and not only to cancer patients, but also to persons suffering from end-stage respiratory, neurological, cardiovascular, AIDS, Alzheimer's Disease, cystic fibrosis, or other life-threatening conditions.

While Hospice primarily provides home care, home care and inpatient care each play an important role, depending upon the needs of the individual patient and family at a particular time.

Hospice views dying as a natural part of life. Hospice does not prolong the dying process or shorten life. When nothing more can be done to cure the disease, Hospice providers give supportive care, addressing the total needs of the dying and those whose lives they touch.

Hospice services are available 7 days a week, 24 hours a day, and are provided by an interdisciplinary team working together to create an atmosphere in which the patient and the family can experience life as fully as possible until the moment of death.

Hospice also provides extended care to support grieving family members and significant others before and during bereavement, for at least thirteen months after the patient's death.

The goals of the Hospice program are several:

1. Help patients live with dignity, each moment of every day, for whatever time they have left.

2. Keep the patients free from pain, as well as free from the fear of anticipatory pain, in relation to their illness. (This pain can be not only physical, but also emotional, social, spiritual, financial, or legal pain, and can affect the family and significant others as well as the patient.)

3. Help the families and significant others participate in the caregiving process, living each moment of each day to the fullest.

4. Provide bereavement support to help families resolve their grief and rebuild their lives.

5. Provide community education programs that present alternatives to conventional curative care for those who are terminally ill and educate the medical community to encourage the acceptance of Hospice/palliative care into mainstream medicine.

Reference

Brochure (Westbury, NY: Long Island Foundation for Hospice Care and Research, Inc., 1985).

Q: What is the history of Hospice? How did it start?

Institutions dedicated to the care of the dying have existed for more than 2,000 years. The term Hospice comes from the Middle Ages, when travelers were given hospitality on their journey. It was a welcoming place for the weary travelers. The words hospital, *hostel*, and *hospice* were used interchangeably. Later, as functions gradually became more specialized, they became terms for separate institutions.

The modern Hospice movement was founded by Dame Cicely Saunders, M.D., in 1967, with the opening of St. Christopher's Hospice in Sydenham, near London, England, with the emphasis on symptom control and on dying as a natural process. Dr. Saunders emphasized the need for effective symptom control, care of the patient and family as a unit, an interdisciplinary approach, the use of volunteers, a continuum of care including home care, continuity of care across different settings, and follow-up of the family members after the patient's death.

Based on Dr. Saunders's work, the first Hospice in the United States was established as Hospice, Inc., in New Haven, Connecticut. As a home care agency, the first patient was accepted in 1974. Planning was begun to create an environment for Hospice patients who could not remain at home. The program grew to become the Connecticut Hospice, Inc., and in 1980 a 44-bed inpatient Hospice facility was opened in Branford, Connecticut.

In 1975, the second American Hospice program was the Hospice at St. Luke's Hospital in New York City. This program was a uniquely American adaptation, the "inpatient scattered-bed consultative model."

At St. Luke's, beds in the hospital were made available to the Hospice patient as needed, and the plan of care was developed with primary consultation with the patient's attending physician and the St. Luke's hospital staff.

New Hospice groups began forming, and great strides were made in Hospice program activities all across the United States. These agencies took various forms, based on locale and other demographics, with patterns expressive of diverse community need and the perception of these needs, the extent of community leadership and financial support, plus resources available in health care, social services, and spiritual care (Amenta and Bohnet, 1988).

There are three major differences in the way Hospices were established in England and the United States. The English Hospice programs were created under the leadership of their physicians and were accepted directly into the medical community. From the beginning, the English Hospices were funded by the National

Health Service and also received community philanthropic support.

In the United States, Hospice programs initially were an outgrowth of an emerging grass roots community-based awareness that the needs of terminally ill patients and their families were not being met by conventional mainstream medical care.

Some physicians were involved, but the Hospice movement was not physician led. In the beginning, programs struggled for financial support and the recognition that Hospice care is a legitimate, viable alternative to conventional curative medical care. Initially, Hospice programs in the United States received financial support only from philanthropic sources.

A campaign to gain continuing federal reimbursement legislation for all Hospice care culminated in August 1982. This was an optional Hospice benefit for people who were eligible for Medicare and was passed as part of the Tax Equity and Fiscal Responsibility Act (TEFRA). The final regulations appeared in the *Federal Register* on December 16, 1983 (Amenta and Bohnet, 1988).

The modern Hospice is now in its third decade.* The National Hospice Organization estimates, in their "NHO Newsletter" (August 1991) that

> There were 1,874 planned or operational hospices in the U.S. at the end of 1991. Hospice remains the fastest growing segment of the health care industry, with an annual growth rate of 12 percent. [These numbers include about 1,831 operational Hospice programs and 43 programs in the planning stage.]
>
> Approximately 96 percent of all hospices are nonprofit organizations. This includes religious and government organizations.

---

* Effective November 1, 1983, Hospice care became a benefit provided through Medicare, Section 1861 (u) of the Social Security Act. Conditions of Participation are set forth in 42 CFR Part 418.42. CFR 418.100 is an additional condition applicable only to Hospices that provide short-term inpatient care and respite *directly* rather than through contractual arrangements. Section 1866 (a) (1) (Q) of the Act as added by 4206 (a) (1) (C) of the Omnibus Budget Reconciliation Act of 1990, Public Law Number 101-508 requires Hospices to file an agreement with the Secretary to comply with the requirements found in Section 1866 of the Act regarding *advance directives*.

Approximately 1,100 [or two of every three] hospice programs are Medicare certified, and more are pending certification.

By comparison, in "Hospice Fact Sheet" (October 10, 1995), the NHO states:

. . . As of August 31, 1995, the NHO has knowledge of 2,544 operational or planned hospice programs in all 50 states and Puerto Rico. In the 1990s annual growth of new hospices has averaged about eight percent.

. . . Approximately 74 percent of hospices are non-profit; four percent are government organizations [federal, state, or local]; 12 percent are for-profit; and 10 percent are "other" or unidentified.

A number of other organizations have come into being, focused on providing information, education, training, and support, both for the professionals and volunteers involved in Hospice care as well as for terminally ill patients and families seeking help, guidance, and referrals. Some of these agencies are listed in Chapter 12.

As the Hospice movement continued to expand, more and more Hospice physicians realized it was important for them to take a leadership role. In 1988, the Academy of Hospice Physicians was created. In 1996, this organization changed its name to the American Academy of Hospice and Palliative Medicine. An international group, its members and

. . . governing board are physicians who wanted a unique forum for discussion and education in the complicated care of the terminally ill. Its goal is to establish Hospice Medicine as an organized medical discipline and an important component of the health care delivery system.

With over 1,500 members representing more than 30 specialties [as of November, 1995], the Academy is dedicated to providing education, research and support for physicians who participate in the management of the care of the terminally ill.

The academy offers physicians a forum for debate and education on the ethical and moral issues related to terminal care "...as part of their involvement in the hospice/palliative approach to patient care and commitment to the improvement of the care of the dying."

These enlightened physicians recognize that death is not "the enemy," nor is it a failure of their professional skills. More and more physicians encourage and promote patient autonomy and recognize that ". . .the proper role of the physician is to help the sick, even when cure is not possible."

"The Academy recognizes that death is a natural and inevitable end to life, and that helping patients achieve an appropriate and easy passage to death is one of the most important and rewarding services that a physician can provide."

They believe that

...physicians have an important responsibility in hospice/palliative care and, through education, research and training, should take a leadership role in promoting and guiding the future direction of this care.

The Academy believes that physicians have a major responsibility for bringing the hospice approach into mainstream medicine and eliminating the dichotomy whereby patients receive either curative or palliative care.

Nurses, social workers, clergy, administrators, volunteers, attorneys, community leaders, and some of our more enlightened political leaders have long been involved in helping the Hospice movement come into its own in the United States. Now, with the active involvement of Hospice physicians, together with caring physicians from other medical disciplines, we can be assured of the future of quality Hospice/palliative care in the United States.

(See also Chapter 7, "American Academy of Hospice and Palliative Medicine.")

References

Amenta, M., and N. Bohnet, *Nursing Care of the Terminally Ill* (Boston: Little, Brown & Company, 1988).

Brochure (St. Petersburg, FL: Academy of Hospice Physicians, 1991).

Smith, Dale C., Exec. Dir., Academy of Hospice Physicians (Gainesville, FL: Private communication, November, 1995).

B. GENERAL

1. What are the admission criteria for a Hospice patient?
2. What is meant by availability of Hospice services?
3. What are definitions of services that the Hospice will provide to the patient and family?
4. What are the objectives of Hospice care?
5. Which Hospice services are covered by some private insurance companies?
6. Are there different types of Hospice programs?
7. Is there a difference in the way Medicare certified Hospices offer their services, even if they are in the same area and serve the same patient population?
8. Who pays for the services provided by Hospice programs?
9. What are the financial costs of Hospice care for Hospice patients and their families?
10. Do the patients and families give up hope when they are admitted to Hospice ?
11. What is meant by "quality assurance" in the Hospice program?
12. Disposal of controlled drugs: What happens to the unused medication(s) in the home when the physician changes the prescription or the patient dies?
13. How will the spiritual needs of patients, families, and significant others be met by the Hospice program? How does Hospice handle the spiritual needs of an atheist or a metaphysician?
14. What is "unfinished business"?

Q: What are the admission criteria for a Hospice patient?

Hospice programs have established criteria for admission to be used when assessing patient referrals to the Hospice program.

1. The patient's illness is in the final stages, with a life expectancy of six months or less.
2. Only palliative care (supportive comfort care) is deemed most appropriate; neither definitive curative treatment nor measures to prolong life beyond its natural end are indicated or sought after by the patient and his or her physician.
3. There is at least one willing, supportive person (primary care person) to be responsible for providing care to the patient in the home.

4. The patient resides in the Hospice service area. A general guideline for distance will be approximately one hour travel time from the Hospice office to the patient's home.

5. The patient's attending physician certifies the prognosis of six months or less and consents to and authorizes Hospice care for the patient.

6. The patient and family are fully informed and give their consent to participation in the Hospice program. When a patient is unable to give informed consent, his or her legal representative may do so on his or her behalf.

7. The patient and the attending physician agree to use a Hospice-affiliated hospital (or nursing home) for inpatient care.

Patient/families will be admitted to Hospice based on these criteria *and* dependent on Hospice's ability to serve them.

Q: What is meant by availability of Hospice services?

The services of Hospice are available on a 24 hours a day / 7 days a week basis consistent with state and federal regulations. Home health nursing, physician care, and drugs/biologicals are routinely available on a 24-hour basis. A nurse or social worker is on duty during nonbusiness weekday hours, weekends, and holidays. The person on call is accessed through a centralized answering service that contacts her or him by phone or beeper. He or she is responsible for the direct provision of home nursing care and the coordination of other services as needed. Administrative and supervisory personnel are available for consultation. Physician care is normally provided in all settings by the patient's attending physician or other physicians with whom arrangements have been established. The Hospice medical director is available to provide direct care to the extent that these needs are not met by the attending physicians. Drugs and biologicals are available during irregular hours through Hospice's network of pharmacies that have pharmacists available at all times for emergency dispensing of medications. A patient needing inpatient care may be admitted to a contract facility where there is an available designated bed in accordance with established Hospice policies and procedures.

All required services other than those mentioned above are available on a 24-hour basis to the extent necessary to meet the needs of individuals for care that is reasonable and necessary for the palliation and management of terminal illness and related conditions. During the process of developing, reviewing, and revising individual patient care plans, the amount and the schedule of hours for any needed services is specified. The means of providing any particular service also is specified. Emergency needs for non-routine services are addressed through the patient care (nurse) coordinator or on-call nurse.

The possible services covered under a patient's care plan are: home care nursing, social work services, physician care, dietary counseling, pastoral care, psycho/social counseling, short-term inpatient care for symptom management or respite, medical appliances and supplies including drugs and biologicals, home health aide/personal care/homemaker/housekeeper services, physical therapy, occupational therapy, speech-language pathology services, audiology, respiratory therapy, laboratory, bereavement care, and volunteer support services, plus financial and legal guidance.

Q: What are definitions of services that the Hospice will provide to the patient and family?

To avoid semantic misunderstandings, it is important to define the services provided in the Hospice program. These services include:

Case Management: Coordination of care through interdisciplinary planning is conducted by the patient care (nurse) coordinator, medical director, social worker and pastoral counselor in conjunction with other caregivers, particularly the attending physician.

Home Health Nursing: Registered nurses provide skilled care through periodic visitation or on a continuous basis as medically necessary.

Physician Services: The patient's attending physician provides her or his medical care. The services of other physicians, including the Hospice medical director, are arranged through the Hospice as needed.

Pastoral Care: The pastoral caregiver(s) or clergy are designated by the patient and family and integrated into the care team. The pastoral counselor coordinates the services of designated pastoral caregiver(s) or clergy and provides spiritual and supportive counseling as needed.

Social Work: Various types of psychosocial intervention and case-work services are provided by the social worker.

Specialty Therapies: Dietary counseling, physical therapy, occupational therapy, speech/language pathology, audiology, respiratory therapy are available as needs indicate.

Counseling: Assistance in adjusting to severe illness, dying, death, and bereavement are available through the social worker, nurse, pastoral counselor, and dietary counselor, as well as other skilled staff. Referrals may be made to community professionals for extensive or in-depth counseling.

Paraprofessional Services: Home health aides, personal care workers, housekeepers, and homemakers are available as needed and are under the supervision of a registered nurse.

Volunteer Support Services: Certified volunteers who have received the required hours of training (which may differ for individual programs) provide emotional support to patients and their families. They may also offer other helping services and practical support as requested by families.

Medically Related Goods and Support Services: Pharmaceutical services, laboratory services, supplies, equipment, and appliances are arranged for as needed.

Inpatient Services: Admission to an affiliated community hospital may be needed for acute attention to the management of symptoms. Respite inpatient care is available for short stays in an affiliated hospital or nursing home.

Bereavement Care: A supportive relationship with family members and significant others of the patient is maintained, usually up to thirteen months after death. The family can request further bereavement support after this period. Various members of the care teams are involved in bereavement care, which is coordinated by the bereavement coordinator.

Q: What are the objectives of Hospice care?

The objectives of Hospice care are:

* Define the terminally ill person and his or her family as the unit of care.
* Involve the terminally ill person and his or her family as part of the care planning team, allowing them to retain final say in decision making concerning care.

- Provide a professional interdisciplinary care planning team comprised of nurse, physician, social worker, pastoral counselor, and nutritionist, who plan care in cooperation with the terminally ill person and his or her family.
- Make available nursing, medical, pastoral, and social work services seven days a week, twenty-four hours a day.
- Make available specially trained volunteers as well as physical therapy, occupational therapy and speech therapy services, and other services as needed.
- Maintain central administration and record keeping.
- Focus on care in the home when this is feasible and desired by the terminally ill person and his or her family. Coordinate inpatient care when necessary.
- Maintain continuity of services wherever the terminally ill person is cared for (at home, in an institution, or in a special residential facility).
- Maintain appropriately high staff-to-patient ratio whether home care or inpatient service.
- Provide symptomatic relief of the terminally ill person's physical distress/symptoms.
- Make counseling available.
- Maintain open, direct, and honest communication with the terminally ill person and his or her family.

Q: Which Hospice services are covered by private insurance companies?

Private insurance coverage for Hospice services may vary, depending on the individual contract. One example is the private insurance coverage offered by Empire Blue Cross and Blue Shield of New York, as follows:

HOSPICE CARE: Up to 210 days of in-patient Hospice care is available in a Hospice or hospital and home care and out-patient services described below provided by the Hospice as long as:

a) the Member has been certified by his primary attending physician as having a life expectancy of six (6) months or less; and

b) the Hospice care is provided by a Hospice organization certified pursuant to Article 40 of the New York Public Health Law; or if the Hospice is located outside of this state, under a

similar certification process required by the state in which the
Hospice organization is located.

Covered Hospice care and out-patient services typically consist
of:

1. Bed patient care either in a designated Hospice unit or in a
regular hospital bed.
2. Day care services provided by the Hospice organization.
3. Home care and outpatient services which are provided by
the Hospice and for which the Hospice charges you. The services
may include at least the following:
   a. Intermittent care by an R.N., L.P.N. or Home Health
      Aides.
   b. Physical therapy.
   c. Speech therapy.
   d. Occupational therapy.
   e. Respiratory therapy.
   f. Social services.
   g. Nutritional services.
   h. Laboratory examinations, x-rays, chemotherapy and
      radiation therapy when required for control or
      symptoms.
   i. Medical supplies.
   j. Drugs and medications prescribed by a physician and
      which are considered approved under the U.S.
      Pharmacopoeia and/or National Formulary. We will
      not pay when the drug or medication is of an
      experimental nature.
   k. Medical care provided by the Hospice physician.
   l. Five visits for bereavement counseling for the Member's
      family either before or after his death.
   m. Durable medical equipment (rental only).
   n. Transportation between home and hospital or Hospice
      organization when medically necessary.

When the care is by a facility which has an agreement with
this Plan or any other Blue Cross Plan in New York State you
will receive full benefits for covered services. When the facility
does not have such an agreement with us, coverage is limited to

80% of the average payment we would make for a like service to a participating facility.

The benefits provided by this rider shall not be available for more than once during a Member's lifetime.

Other than stated above, there is no change in any of the terms of the Contract and/or Certificate to which this rider is attached.

Q: Are there different types of Hospice programs?

Yes. Hospice programs are different, and it is important to know and understand the kind and extent of the services offered, as well as the organizational structure and how the individual program is reimbursed for its services.

There might be a difference in *legal status*. The program may be incorporated as an independent community-based agency controlled by its own identified governing board, or it may be a division of another corporation and controlled by that parent corporation. It could be a coalition program with leadership from a hospital or a nursing home; or it could derive its leadership from a home health agency, a government agency, or a religious organization.

Hospices may be *voluntary* (with nonprofit ownership and control) or *proprietary* (with private for-profit ownership and control). There may be private nonprofit ownership and control; federal, state, or other government ownership; or religious affiliation with private, nonprofit ownership and control.

Regardless of whether the Hospice is *nonprofit* or *for-profit*, this tax status does not affect the rigorous Medicare certification requirements. All Medicare certified Hospices must abide by the same federal guidelines, including the requirement for volunteers and their recruitment, training, and placement.

Regardless of tax status, a Hospice must meet the community expectations to serve the medically indigent patients based upon need and not inability to pay for services . . . Medicare and other third party payers reimburse [for-profit] Hospices at the same rate as not-for-profit Hospices. Regardless of tax status, a Hospice with a large [patient] census is more cost effective than a Hospice with a small census . . . A Hospice which can achieve economies of scale will have excess revenue over expenses (Parker, 1995).

The Hospice program might be a completely independent, community-based program, limiting its services only to the care of terminally ill persons. Or it might be part of a larger program that serves a wider patient population. The "Hospice Fact Sheet" (October 1995) states,

There is no current mandatory nationwide accreditation or "seal of approval," although many programs are certified voluntarily by Medicare and JCAHO (the Joint Commission on Accreditation of Healthcare Organizations) . . . Hospice is covered by Medicaid in 36 states plus the District of Columbia.

Some states require that Hospice programs be Medicare/Medicaid certified as well as licensed; other states require only licensure. In some cases, there may be informal Hospice-type programs that are not incorporated and operate informally.

". . . Thirty-five states have hospice licensing laws (58 percent of all Hospices are licensed), six have licensure pending, and ten states plus the District of Columbia do not have hospice licensure" ("Hospice Fact Sheet").

There are five major "primary service" types of programs:

1. *Patient-support* programs focus primarily on meeting the non-medical needs of terminally ill patients;

2. *Counseling services* programs generally provide patients and their families psychological support services, including bereavement services;

3. *Inpatient services* programs provide primarily inpatient services for terminally ill patients;

4. *Home health* programs offer services that are targeted to the terminally ill in their homes; and

5. *Complete Hospice* programs offer comprehensive, specialized services for terminally ill patients, their families, and significant others, including patient/family support and bereavement services, and combine home care with inpatient care when needed. Some may also offer residential care on a case-by-case basis.

Hospice programs may be Medicare/Medicaid certified in five major categories: (1) independent, community-based; (2) hospital-based; (3) nursing home-based; (4) home health agency-based; or (5) a free-standing inpatient facility, possibly connected with a home health agency or an independent community-based agency.

In regional areas, two or more Hospice programs may come together, to form an alliance or consortium—to better meet the total needs of the patient, family, and significant others—as well as address Hospice bottom-line (financial) issues.

Some Hospice programs have "multiple Hospice locations" (MHLs). *Not* identified as branch Hospices, the MHLs are administered out of a central office location, but are staffed within the different communities, encouraging greater individual community interest and involvement.

References

Galen Miller, V.P., National Hospice Organization (Arlington, VA: Private Communication, November 1995).

National Hospice Organization, *The 1991 Guide to the Nation's Hospices* (Arlington, VA), p. 15.

_____ "Hospice Fact Sheet" (Arlington, VA: Updated October 10, 1995).

Andrew T. Parker, Partner, American Hospice Management; AHM manages both proprietary and nonprofit Hospices (Bethesda, MD: Private communication, November 1995).

Q: Is there a difference in the way Medicare certified Hospices offer their services, even if they are in the same area and serve the same patient population?

Yes. In one example, a Medicare certified program in a suburban area has a hospital as its parent organization. Both are not-for-profit. This Hospice requires that the patient/family/significant others come directly to the Hospice office as part of the admissions/intake process. If the patient is not able to come (still in the hospital or not able to leave home), then at least one of the family/prospective caregivers must come to the office without the patient.

Another Medicare certified Hospice in the same geographic area, also a not-for-profit agency, is incorporated as an independent community-based program. As part of their admissions/intake process, they will send a Hospice staff person directly to the patient's home or to the hospital if the patient is still in the hospital. Some Medicare certified programs may require signed do-not-resuscitate orders before admission to the program. Other Hospices will accept the patient into the program and then work with the patient and his or her family/significant others to educate them and help them come to an informed decision regarding "advance directives" for the patient's care. (See "How Can the Patient and Family Be Assured Their Wishes Will Be Made Known to the Hospice Team?" in Chapter 6.)

Some Hospices will not accept a patient if there is no primary caregiver at home. Other programs will work with the patient to help create a "primary care system." (See "Why Is Having a Primary Caregiver So Important to the Patient in a Hospice Program?" in Chapter 2.)

According to the National Hospice Organization (1995): "Forty-five percent of Hospices admit patients without primary caregivers; another 31 percent admit patients without caregivers on a case-by-case basis" ("Hospice Fact Sheet").

More and more Hospice programs are extending their bereavement programs to the larger community in general, whether or not the patient, family, and significant others were in the Hospice program. As Hospices become more involved with the community-at-large, these situations may cover death due to trauma or accident, as well as terminal illness.

. . . Hospices work with a wide variety of community organizations in providing bereavement support. Sixty-three percent of Hospices work with churches [and synagogues]; 55 percent work with hospitals; 50 percent with schools; 46 percent with nursing homes; 28 percent provide services and support to community mental health agencies; and 27 percent work with organizations such as Widowed Persons Service, American Cancer Society, and Compassionate Friends. Approximately ten percent of Hospices also provide services and support to police departments, corporations, and anti-drunk driving groups ("Hospice Fact Sheet").

Hospices may also differ in the kind of bereavement services offered in their program. The "Hospice Fact Sheet" states:

> Sixty-nine percent of Hospice patients and families accept bereavement services . . . 80 percent of Hospices provide support group services; 67 percent offer memorial services; 63 percent provide educational programs to the community; 60 percent provide individual/family counseling; 43 percent provide crisis counseling; 35 percent provide specific children's services; and 15 percent provide emergency room support.

References

National Hospice Organization, "Hospice Fact Sheet" (Arlington, VA: Updated October 10, 1995).

Margaret Duncan, Information Referral Coordinator, National Hospice Organization (Arlington, VA: Private Communication, November, 1995).

Galen Miller, V.P., National Hospice Organization (Arlington, VA: Private communication, November 1995).

Q: Who pays for the services provided by Hospice programs?

Reimbursement depends upon the type of program and the services it offers. A Medicare/Medicaid certified program receives reimbursement from Medicare (federal government), Medicaid (federal, state, and local governments), Blue Cross/Blue Shield, and a number of commercial insurers. It contracts with health maintenance organizations (HMOs) and other managed care programs, and charges fees to patients and families according to their ability to pay.

An overview of medical coverage for Hospice services was provided by the National Hospice Organization in 1995 ("Fact Sheet").

> Seventy-five percent of Hospices are either Medicare-certified or pending certification. In 1994 Medicare spent $1.2 billion of its roughly $200 billion budget on Hospice services.

. . . Hospice is covered under Medicaid in 36 states plus the District of Columbia. In 1993 Medicaid spent $129 million on Hospice services.

. . . Coverage for Hospice is provided to more than 80 percent of employees in medium and large businesses. Eighty-two percent of managed care plans offer Hospice services. In addition, most private insurance plans include a Hospice benefit.

. . . In 1995 the Federal Register published the authorization of a Hospice benefit under CHAMPUS (the Civilian Health and Medical Program of the Uniformed Services).

Hospice groups may receive funding from a number of other sources, since reimbursement for services rendered accounts for only about 75-80 percent of the Hospice costs. Note that the government-mandated bereavement care is not reimbursed by Medicare, nor is it a reimbursable service under most third-party payors. However, some states may require partial reimbursement from insurers. For example, New York State mandates coverage for five bereavement visits. A unique component of the Hospice program is that full bereavement services are offered to all patients, their families, and significant others.

Many Hospice programs have expanded their services in community outreach. "Eighty-one percent of Hospices offer bereavement programs and services to the community-at-large, not just those families served directly by Hospice" ("Hospice Fact Sheet").

Financial support from the community is essential for the survival of the programs and may come from various sources, such as government (federal, state, local) grants, corporate and foundation grants, gifts from individuals and groups, bequests and memorial contributions, and proceeds from fundraising projects.

Reference

National Hospice Organization, "Hospice Fact Sheet" (Arlington, VA: Updated October 10, 1995).

Q: What are the financial costs of Hospice care for Hospice patients and their families?

Hospice care is a mix of volunteer and professional services. Many of the professional services are covered by various types of health insurance plans. (See Chapters 1 and 9.) The Hospice social worker is available to discuss your insurance with you so you will receive maximum coverage from your health insurance. Some insurance plans, such as Medicare, Medicaid, some Health Maintenance Organizations and other managed care programs, and many Blue Cross plans, provide very comprehensive coverage with little or no uncovered services. Other insurance plans provide only limited coverage for Hospice care, and some impose restrictions on home care. By reviewing your policy and speaking to your company directly, Hospice will be able to let you know exactly what is covered and what, if anything, will be your responsibility.

After insurance payments are made, should there be an uncovered balance due to Hospice, Hospice staff will discuss this with you and charges will be billed directly to you. However, adjustments may be made, depending on your ability to pay. Should you have any questions about these matters during your involvement with Hospice, a staff member will be glad to discuss them with you.

Special note about drugs and medical supplies. Hospice has the responsibility of coordinating the provision of any drugs or medical supplies that may become necessary at home. This is done via the pharmacies and supply companies with which the Hospice contracts. If you are on Medicare or have an insurance plan that reimburses Hospice directly for these items, Hospice will pay the vendor and collect from the insurance company. Any deductibles or co-payments that apply will be your responsibility. The Medicare Hospice Benefit, for example, has a patient co-payment of $5.00 per prescription or 5 percent per prescription, whichever amount is *lower*. Hospice will bill you for these co-payment amounts. If you are not on Medicare or an insurance plan that reimburses Hospice directly for these items, the pharmacy or supplier will bill you or any applicable insurance directly. These charges then become your responsibility.

Reference

U.S. Dept. of Health and Human Services, Health Care Financing Administration. *Hospice Benefits.* U. S. Govt. Printing Office, 1995, #396-894/00507.

Q: Do the patients and families give up hope when they are admitted to Hospice?

No, patients and families do not give up hope. The hope that is experienced by the patient and family will remain the same, but the *object* of what is hoped for will change. At the beginning of the illness, the patient may hope for a cure. As the terminal condition progresses, the object of hope changes for a remission, then freedom from pain and symptoms.

Hospice does not aim to restore the patient's biological integrity but to assist the patient and family to live as fully as possible for whatever time is left.

Hope becomes an essential ingredient in the plan of care. It is a major component of Hospice contribution to the inner healing process, and for some patients hope becomes an integral part of the dying process.

To be effective, hope—no matter how transient—must be realistic. Spirituality and religion promote hope in that they provide an understanding of illness and mortality, a basis for coping with sickness and suffering.

Death is not the ultimate tragedy of life. The ultimate tragedy of life is depersonalization—dying in an alien and sterile area, separated from the spiritual nourishment that comes from being able to reach out to a loving hand, separated from a desire to experience the things that make life worth living separated from hope (Cousins, 1979).

The challenge of Hospice is to sustain patients in a "personalized" environment, an environment that recognizes individual needs and attempts to reduce individual fears. Without denying death, Hospice philosophy accepts the limitations of brief prognosis to promote maximum physical and psychological comfort. Patients come with no hope of recovery from physical disease, yet full of hope for relief from suffering. Hospice care generates hope in what often appears to be a hopeless situation (O'Connor, 1986).

References

Cousins, N., *Anatomy of an Illness* (New York: Norton, 1979), p. 133.

O'Connor, P., "Spiritual Elements of Hospice Care," *The Hospice Journal* (Summer 1986), 2(2):99-108.

Q: What is meant by "quality assurance" in the Hospice program?

In order to ensure that patients, their families, and significant others are receiving competent and appropriate care, each Hospice has a quality assurance program. The Hospice commitment to the provision of the highest possible quality of patient/family care is implemented through the services of the interdisciplinary team, volunteers, and other staff and by the monitoring and evaluation of the quality, appropriateness, and cost-effectiveness of these services (JCAH, 1983).

In a Hospice program, a quality and appropriateness review refers to activities that ensure quality of clinical care for patients and families and also includes the assessment of the overall program organization and effectiveness (Rolka, 1983).

The Hospice quality assurance committee is charged with the responsibility of overseeing and guiding the development, implementation, and review of these plans, including the conducting of a semi-annual evaluation. The goals are:

1. To conduct an ongoing objective assessment of Hospice services; and

2. To identify, correct, and reevaluate any problems in the operation of the Hospice program (*By-laws*, 1989).

References

By-laws and *Hospice Operations Manual* (Hempstead, NY: Long Island Foundation for Hospice Care and Research, Inc., 1989), pp. 7, 279-90.

Hospice Self-Assessment and Survey Guide (Chicago: Joint Commission on Accreditation of Hospitals [JCAH], 1983), pp. 61-3.

Rolka, H., "Quality Assurance for Terminally Ill," *Hospital and Health Services Administration* (March-April 1983), pp. 66-80.

Q: Disposal of controlled drugs: What happens to the unused medication(s) in the home when the physician changes the prescription or the patient dies?

To prevent the misuse or abuse of physician-prescribed controlled drugs, Hospice programs take action in accordance with accepted standards of practice: controlled drugs listed in FDA Schedules II, III, or IV no longer used by the patient at home are to be properly disposed.

When the patient no longer requires a particular controlled drug, the Hospice nurse will inform the patient/family of the need for destruction of the drug. The nurse, with the concurrence of the family, will dispose of the drug in the home in the presence of another witness (the patient, the primary careperson, or a family member). Documentation reflecting the name and amount of the drug will be prepared at time of disposal and signed by those in attendance. This documentation will become part of the patient's record. In the event the patient or family refuses to destroy the drug(s), the nurse will document that information in the patient's record. (See Appendix A, Figure 1, "Controlled Drug Disposal Record.")

Reference

Hospice Operations Manual (Hempstead, NY: Long Island Foundation for Hospice Care and Research, Inc., 1988), pp. 384-6.

Q: How will the spiritual needs of patients, families, and significant others be met by the Hospice program?

Hospice programs attempt to provide holistic care to persons nearing the end of their lifespan. Holistic care involves an awareness of the complete needs of the total person, including economic needs as well as physical, emotional, and spiritual needs.

The spiritual needs of patients and families/significant others ought not to be confused with religious application. "The terms 'religious care' and 'spiritual care' are frequently used synonymously. Perhaps religious care is spiritual care, but spiritual care is not necessarily religious care" (O'Connor, 1988).

Patients and families have their own spiritual beliefs, and awareness and appreciation of a patient's individual spiritual orientation is essential to holistic care. Therefore the role of the Hospice program is to create an environment where the patient's spiritual orientation can flourish. Sister Anne Munley contends that an effective Hospice team can meet the spiritual needs of patients, families, and significant others and need not be sponsored by a religious organization when caregivers are sensitive to the religious orientation of patients and family; the staff is given continuing education in rituals and practices of various religions; and there is easy access to clergy and sacred rites.

Patients may have strong affiliations with religious institutions. Effort to continue this connection is important. Religious affiliation may hinder or foster attention to spiritual issues. In Hospice care, the needs of the patient dictate the role of the clergy, not the other way around.

In order to enhance quality of life for patients, it is essential that the Hospice evaluate the strengths and resources of each patient to enable him to participate in meeting his own spiritual needs based on his life's patterns of behavior. A Hospice program does not have to know much about different religions or forms of spirituality, but it must have the ability to create an environment whereby the patient's own spiritual growth may continue to occur.

Munley further states that the essence of spiritual caregiving is not doctrine or dogma, but the capacity to enter into the world of others and respond with feeling. This fundamental human capacity involves touching another at a level that is deeper than ideological or doctrinal differences.

> Spiritual issues may include nurturing of the soul, the solace from religious traditions . . . [and] need to be addressed when reviewing the patient's total plan of care and always reflective of the individual's spiritual orientation.

> . . . Patient and families are in a vulnerable state at the time of a terminal illness. The rejection of a clergy person may be perceived as a rejection of God. But it is the needs of the patient that dictate the role of the clergy and not the other way around.

> . . . The evaluation of a patient's spiritual orientation is appropriate in order to diagnose spiritual pain. With spiritual pain one cannot simply point a finger to exactly where it hurts. As with

physical pain, that changes over the course of time, so spiritual pain may change and need to be assessed continuously. Spiritual pain represents the agony of unmet need. Still, it is crucial to realize that the dying process may raise spiritual issues, but not necessarily spiritual pain (O'Connor, 1988).

How does Hospice handle the spiritual needs of an atheist or a metaphysician?

First we listen carefully for verbal and non-verbal messages that may indicate the patient's feelings. A statement such as, "I do not believe in God," may reveal a strong sense of belief in a Universal Source, while for another patient it may convey a special plea for help in facing adversity. Hospice values stress the individual needs of patients. "We do not want patients to think the way we are thinking, we want them to think more deeply in their own way" (O'Connor, 1986).

In conclusion:

Spiritual care for both patients and families is another necessary part of any bona fide Hospice program. All persons approaching their deaths in a conscious and forthright way deserve the opportunity to examine the dimensions of meaning, relatedness, forgiveness, and transcendence that this powerful life event inevitably brings to the fore (Amenta and Bohnet, 1986).

References

Amenta, M., and N. Bohnet, *Nursing Care of the Terminally Ill* (Boston: Little, Brown & Company, 1986), p. 50.

Munley, A., *The Hospice Alternative* (New York: Basic Books, 1983).

O'Connor, P., "The Role of Spiritual Care in Hospice," *The American Journal of Hospice Care* (July/August, 1988), 88:31-7; "Spiritual Elements of Hospice Care." *The Hospice Journal* (Summer 1986), 2(2):99-108.

Saunders, C., "Living with the Dying," *Radiography* (1983), 49:79-83.

Q: What is "unfinished business"?

With the terminal diagnosis and limited prognosis, Hospice caregivers can help their patients, families, and significant others realize that they have been given "a gift of time."

Frequently we are frugal and save for a rainy day; now, it is pouring outside. We are being deluged by the heightened trauma, our reactions to the reality of what is happening to our loved ones, and the dynamics of our family situation. With our new awareness, we now can "seize the moment" and live in the here and now.

Viktor Frankl (a psychiatrist who survived the Auschwitz concentration camp) has said that the last of the human freedoms is not a freedom from pain but the freedom left to choose our response in the given circumstance.

Now, with our increased awareness and sensitivity, we can use this opportunity to complete our "unfinished business." We can take this time to make amends for the things we said and did, or did not do. We can say and do the things we wanted to do but didn't give ourselves time to do.

We can say, "I'm sorry," "Please forgive me," "I love you," "Please let me help you," "Let me be here for you," and so forth. We can open ourselves to give and receive hugs. We can open our hearts and listen—to each other, to the meaning behind our words, to body language, and to our unspoken words.

We can take that pleasure trip for which we were saving. We can learn to accept each other and ourselves just as we are and not be judgmental.

And we can take this critical time to address the more mundane issues involved in putting our "house" in order—including financial and legal matters as well as personal relationships (Sendor, 1992).

Some families will be able to take care of unfinished business, whereas others will not. Some will be able to say their last goodbyes, will be able to plan for the funeral service, and, to a limited extent, discuss the future together. In other families, the patient will die without ever having talked about it openly. And for many patients and their families, this is their need, their way of maintaining family integrity, their style.

Hospice can extend and respond to the invitation to engage in open communication if that will be helpful. But the choice and the decision belong to families alone (Amenta and Bohnet, 1986).

References

Amenta, M., and N. Bohnet, *Nursing Care of the Terminally Ill* (Boston: Little, Brown & Company, 1986), pp. 109, 189.

Sendor, V.F., Presentation to People with AIDS. Long Island: Ayur-Veda Resources of New York, September 19, 1992.

2
PATIENT/FAMILY

1. What is a patient and family bill of rights?

2. What is meant by "Informed Consent"? How is this documented?

3. What happens to the rights of minor patients? What happens to the rights of the incompetent patient?

4. What are the benefits of Hospice services for the family?

5. Will the Hospice permit the family to participate in caring for the patient?

6. Can Hospice assist the patient and family before the patient is medically ready to be admitted to the Hospice program?

7. Why is having a primary caregiver so important to the patient in a Hospice program?

8. Will the Hospice be available to the patient and family whenever they need Hospice services?

9. How can Hospice help family/caregiver(s) who are stressed out and cannot cope?

10. What are the needs of the terminally ill patient and family for intimacy and sexuality?

11. What are some of the things a patient and family might do to maximize the time that is left?

12. Under what circumstances is a Hospice patient transferred from the home to inpatient care in a hospital (or in a nursing home)?

13. What will happen to Hospice patients if they are transferred from care in the home to care in the hospital or nursing home?

14. Will the hospital staff or nursing home staff be knowledgeable in Hospice care?

15. Do Hospice patients ever receive treatments such as surgery, radiation, or chemotherapy?

16. What happens to the patients in the Hospice program if their health care benefits are exhausted?

17. What if the patient and/or family is not pleased with some services or personnel from the Hospice?

18. Will there be confidentiality regarding the patient's medical records and access to the patient's home?

19. Is there ever a time when a patient will be discharged from the Hospice program?

20. What happens when a patient dies at home? What does the family do?

Q: What is a patient and family bill of rights?

Hospice programs have a "patient bill of rights" that will be shared with the patient and family at the time of admission. The patient, family, and significant others will be given the opportunity to discuss these rights with a Hospice staff person for clarification. A written acknowledgment will be obtained from the patient/family and kept in the medical records.

Patient Bill of Rights

1. The right to be listened to and treated as a person.
2. The right to be told the facts concerning my medical condition and to have my questions answered honestly.
3. The right to participate in the decision-making concerning my life and my own treatment.
4. The right to be informed of my rights, my options, the services that Hospice provides, the charges and fees for services, and the name and function of anyone or any agency that provides services to me and my family.
5. The right to a life of quality, as free from pain as possible.
6. The right to have my own lifestyle and values respected, including the sanctity of my body after death.
7. The right to die in peace and dignity, and not to die alone.
8. The right to receive adequate and appropriate care, where and when it is needed.
9. The right to be cared for by sensitive, knowledgeable people and to receive comfort when cure is no longer feasible.
10. The right to expect that the concerns and needs of my family will be acknowledged.
11. The right to refuse to participate in experimental research and to refuse medication and treatment after being fully informed of and understanding the consequences of such actions.

12. The right to have my patient/family records kept confidential, and the right to approve or refuse their release to anyone outside Hospice (except in the case of my transfer to a health facility or as required by law or third-party payor).

13. The right to voice complaints to the New York State Health Department.

14. The right to recommend changes in policies and services of Hospice staff, to the area office representative of the Department of Health or to any outside representative of the patient's choice, free from restraint, interference, coercion, discrimination, or reprisal.

Reference

Hospice Operations Manual (Hempstead, NY: Long Island Foundation for Hospice Care and Research, Inc., 1990), p. 9.

Q: What is meant by "Informed Consent"? How is this documented?

An informed consent is a written indication that the patient and family understand the conditions of the agreement between themselves and the Hospice program. This consent defines the role and responsibility of each in the areas of fully understanding the services of Hospice, the responsibilities of the patient and family, and the financial obligations of each party. See Appendix A, Figure 2, for an example of a Hospice informed consent form.

Reference

Hospice Operations Manual (Hempstead, NY: Long Island Foundation for Hospice Care and Research, Inc., 1990), pp. 332-3.

Q: What happens to the rights of minor patients? What happens to the rights of the incompetent patient?

Rights of the Incompetent Patient

The Hospice will assist the family . . . "to transfer the rights of patients who are judged incompetent to an individual (or committee of individuals) legally authorized to act on behalf of the patient. Hospice recognizes that incompetent patients may at times be capable of making choices about certain aspects of their care. With consent of the individual (or committee of individuals) legally authorized to act on behalf of the patient, such patient choices shall be reflected in the Hospice plan of care.

"If, after admission to the program, an eligible individual who was incompetent at the time of admission thereafter regains competency [the patient has] the right to withdraw from the Hospice program, if so desired."

Rights of Minor Patients

"The rights of a minor patient may be exercised by person(s) legally authorized to act on behalf of the minor patient. Hospice recognizes that minors are often able and desirous of making choices about their care. Therefore a minor patient shall be considered an active member of the Hospice team . . . " and will be invited to take an active part in the development of the individual plan of care.

Reference

Hospice Operations Manual (Hempstead, NY: Long Island Foundation for Hospice Care and Research, Inc., 1990), pp. 329, 331.

Q: What are the benefits of Hospice services for the family?

Hospice encourages the family members to participate in the care of the terminally ill person, with appropriate teaching and guidance. The Hospice team will encourage open communication of information and feelings among family members before and after death of the family member. Hospice also will provide an educational packet to the family to assist them in understanding the dying process. Although Hospice will offer bereavement services to the family for up to thirteen months following the death of the patient, the family can request additional bereavement support, and it will be provided.

Q: Will the Hospice permit the family to participate in caring for the patient?

In addition to encouraging the family as well as the patient, the Hospice will actively involve them in the care planning process. The patient and family will be encouraged to participate in the treatment process. Education and training will be offered to the patient and family about what is happening, what is likely to happen, the processes of dying and grieving, and how they can participate in the implementation of the comprehensive plan of care. Particular emphasis will be placed on comfort measures that can be employed to enhance the quality of life for whatever time is left.

Q: Can Hospice assist the patient and family before the patient is medically ready to be admitted to the Hospice program?

Yes. An assigned Hospice staff person will make an appointment to explain what options and resources are available to the patient, the family, and significant others before the patient is medically ready to be admitted into the Hospice program.

With up-to-date information and alternatives explained, the patient and family become informed medical consumers. This advanced planning prior to the time that the patient becomes terminally ill can be of great help in demystifying the terminal stage of illness. When realistic expectations are made known, the future will be less fearful and the patient/family unit can focus on the "gift of time" that has been given to them to take care of any "unfinished business" and enhance the quality of their lives in whatever way possible and natural for them.

(See "What is 'Unfinished Business'?" in Chapter 1.)

Q: Why is having a primary caregiver so important to the patient in a Hospice program?

Many Hospices will not accept a patient without a primary caregiver (or support system) available in the home. Although Hospice is an intermittent care program, it is responsible for the total plan and program of care for each patient and family. However, Hospice "cannot assume responsibility for the safety of patients who are living outside the supervision and control of Hospice" (Kilburn, 1988) or do not have someone to help them at home. (Note: an exception to intermittent care is the "continuous care" component of Hospice, which is only available under strict symptom-control guidelines.)

An important part of the Hospice philosophy is to involve family members and significant others in the care of the patient by providing the appropriate instruction and training needed to help manage symptoms at home. Also, the "unit of care" is the patient, and family, and significant others. However, there are times when Hospice care is needed and appropriate but a primary caregiver is not available at the time of inquiry.

For example: A frail elderly person may be living alone. Another person may not have a safe home environment (i.e., a dysfunctional family situation) or may have family members who either choose not to care for the patient at home or may not be able to, perhaps because of psychological, emotional, or economic reasons. Perhaps there is another ill family member at home, space limitations, or all family members must work outside the home. Perhaps there is an elderly couple with one spouse who is terminally ill and another who is also ill and not able to cope with the situation due to physical, emotional, or financial limitations.

Faced with this reality, Hospices have become more flexible in defining "primary caregiver." Some Hospices will work with a cooperative candidate for admission, by investigating a "primary care support system," and assisting with arrangement for a safe "home" environment and adequate care. It is important for the patient to be comfortable with both this arrangement, and with the committed people involved who are sharing the caregiving responsibilities.

Various arrangements might be made. As part of this support system, Hospice volunteers could visit on a regular or shift basis; Hospice home health aides or personal care workers could be assigned; nurses, homemakers, and other assistants could be purchased by the patient/family from private funds, or be available through other insurance. A volunteer Hospice "host" family might take a Hospice patient into its home, or move in to care for the Hospice patient in the home of the patient; they "adopt" the patient. Special grant funding might be available to purchase a live-in companion. Special Hospice residences, or alternative community residences or group homes might exist, with Hospice providing care and the residence accepting the primary caregiver role.

Perhaps relatives (other than the immediate family) or neighbors, a religious group, a local college, a community organization, or a nursing home might help with cooperative arrangements.

In most cases, if a system or network for primary caregiving cannot be arranged, the patient will be referred to more appropriate care settings.

References

Kilburn, L. H., *Hospice Operations Manual* (Arlington, VA: National Hospice Organization, 1988), p. 467.

Long Island Foundation for Hospice Care and Research, Inc., *Certificate of Need Application to the Department of Health, New York State, for the Establishment of a Certified Hospice Program* (Hempstead, NY: Revised October 1987), pp. 6-7.

Q: Will the Hospice be available to the patient and family whenever they need Hospice services?

The assigned Hospice staff will be available (on call) to the patient and family twenty-four hours a day, seven days a week, to arrange services and provide supportive care to patients, families, and significant others. The person on call will respond to such calls by telephone to assess the need and make a follow-up home visit, if necessary.

Q: How can Hospice help family/caregiver(s) who are stressed out and canot cope?

Hospice can provide compassionate understanding and special support services for the family/caregiver(s) who are stressed out and cannot cope.

The fact and the reality of both the diagnosis and the terminal prognosis are difficult enough. Added to the initial shock may be a drain on financial resources, the complexity of the process involved in applying for health care benefits, and the emotional strain on interpersonal relationships and family dynamics.

There may be confusion and differences of opinion—among family members and the caregiver(s) and even between the patient and the family—as to *what* to do about the care of the patient, *how* to do it, and *when*.

The Hospice program recognizes this potential for added stress. Built into the Hospice admission process are carefully considered steps. The admissions staff person carefully explains exactly what Hospice is, what the program can provide, and what it does *not* do. Patient/family rights, responsibilities, and advance directives are reviewed. The patient and family are invited to become part of the interdisciplinary team, with invaluable input into the creation, implementation, and review of the patient/family plan of care.

Volunteers may be assigned to a particular family to help. Home health aides, homemakers, and members of the team also will be assigned. The nurse and social worker work with the patient's primary physician. A clergy person, nutritionist, or various therapists may be assigned to provide spiritual and other support services.

The plan of care may include some respite time for the patient in a hospital or nursing home. This usually is done to monitor pain control and symptom management and can be coordinated with the instruction and training of family members and significant others, so they can do their part in the care of the patient at home. Thus, the patient is able to come to a safe home environment.

The delivery of some special equipment and supplies will have taken place. An individualized schedule will have been arranged. The caregiver(s) will know how and when to administer any necessary medications. They will be shown how to bathe and feed and toilet the patient. They will be taught how to observe, listen, and report changes in the patient's condition to the assigned members of the interdisciplinary team.

Caregivers do become tired, even with all the team support, and there may come a time when families, caregivers, and significant others, even in the most caring and loving families, just cannot cope any longer.

As the patient's condition lingers, worsens, or requires more intensive care, there may be patient personality changes. Family caregivers may be experiencing heightened trauma and sleep deprivation. It becomes difficult for them to recognize and take care of their own needs. They may not be able to cope with the "normal" daily activities for themselves and other family members (if any). They may "get in their own way" and not be able to help with the patient's needs. They may feel inadequate, frustrated, and in despair.

The Hospice interdisciplinary team can arrange for respite "time-off." Perhaps additional volunteers may be assigned. Compassionate listening can help get to the root of the problem(s) and help address the real issues. "Anticipatory Grief" symptoms may be recognized. (See also "What is 'Anticipatory Grief'?" in Chapter 11.) The patient may be transferred to an inpatient unit for a few days (maximum is usually five days) so the caregiver(s) can address the issue of "What about my needs!"—be able to identify them *and* take care of them. They may be encouraged to go away for a few days, take care of personal chores, or visit with friends and neighbors—or other family members. When the patient returns home, the situation will be carefully monitored and help offered that is appropriate and timely.

Sometimes it may be difficult for the caregiver(s) to cope with the situation at home when death is imminent. Although philosophically and ideally it is better to keep the patient at home, it may be necessary to transfer the patient to a hospital for the end-stage of the dying process. Whatever changes are made in the plan of care, the "unit of care" remains the patient, the family, and significant others, and any changes will reflect this, to enhance the quality of their lives in positive and life-affirming ways.

Q: What are the needs of the terminally ill patient and family for intimacy and sexuality?

Just because the patient is terminally ill, patterns of a lifetime do not change in importance. The patient may express the method of meeting needs for intimacy in a different manner. The family, with the starting of anticipatory grief, may feel that it is not appropriate to discuss these issues of intimacy and sexuality with the patient. Since this is a most precious time for all concerned, it is important that these issues and concerns be addressed.

The appropriate member of the Hospice team will assist the patient and family, as a unit, in realizing that sexuality and the need for intimacy is not a forbidden subject and will encourage the expression of love and affection to continue in the patient's pattern of a lifetime.

Q: What are some of the things a patient and family might do to maximize the time that is left?

The time that remains can be used for the benefit of both the patient and the family. This can be a "Time of Remembering," whereby the patient can tell his or her life story and leave a living legacy for future generations. This can be done in many ways, and always, each patient's wishes must be respected.

Perhaps a home video could be created and the patient's story enhanced by the addition of favorite music and photographs at appropriate intervals. Since some patients may not want to be rememberd looking so ill, perhaps an audiotape could be made, so just the patient's voice can be heard communicating with the family and sharing a life story. Writing in a daily diary or journal, or putting together a photo album are other ways to record a life story. A trunk of favorite mementos and correspondence can be invaluable, too.

Q: Under what circumstances is a Hospice patient transferred from the home to inpatient care in a hospital (or in a nursing home)?

There are certain times and conditions when it would be appropriate for a Hospice patient to be admitted for inpatient care: for 24-hour monitoring of pain and symptom control when this cannot be done at home; to provide respite care for five days for the family, when this would assist the family in creating a better home environment by providing family teaching to care for the patient at home, or to give the family some needed respite time-off due to the stress and trauma of caring for the patient. Or perhaps certain circumstances arise where it is considered best for all for the patient to be transferred to the hospital as death becomes imminent.

Q: What will happen to Hospice patients if they are transferred from care in the home to care in the hospital or nursing home?

When a Hospice patient is admitted to the hospital (or nursing home) for appropriate backup inpatient care, a copy of the current, specific plan of care will be issued to the inpatient staff within 24 hours of admission. The Hospice will monitor the review of inpatient care. The purpose of these reviews is to ensure that the patient's care in the hospital or nursing home is in compliance with the Hospice concept and the patient's plan of care. During the inpatient stay, the Hospice staff will be available to the patient and family as well as available for consultation to the inpatient staff. The hospital staff assigned to provide care for the Hospice patient are considered members of the Hospice interdisciplinary team providing direct input that could affect the plan of care.

Q: Will the hospital staff or nursing home staff be knowledgeable in Hospice care ?

Hospice programs have contractual agreements with certain hospitals and nursing homes for the admission of their Hospice patients. As part of these agreements, the Hospice will conduct inservice education for the hospital and nursing home staff on all the units containing designated Hospice beds. Inservice or support meetings may be requested by the hospital or nursing home staff at any time to ensure continuity of care for Hospice patients while they are in the hospital or nursing home.

Q: Do Hospice patients ever receive treatments such as surgery, radiation, or chemotherapy?

Yes. Hospice patients may undergo certain surgical procedures if they are related to the comfort-care of the patient and will help control adverse symptoms. The attending physician or Hospice medical director may recommend disease-specific therapy such as palliative chemotherapy, palliative radiation, or certain limited surgical procedures to help control pain and better manage specific symptoms.

Q: What happens to the patients in the Hospice program if their health care benefits are exhausted?

Hospice programs, once they have admitted a patient, will not discharge the patient/family or diminish the quality or level of services because of exhaustion of health care insurance benefits. If no substitute, supplementary, or complementary method of reimbursement is available to the patient/family, the Hospice will bill the patient/family for services rendered, with fees based on the existing per visit charge and the patient/family's ability to pay. If no funds are available and the patient/family have exhausted all options, the Hospice will absorb the cost of care provided to the patient/family.

Q: What if the patient and/or family is not pleased with some services or personnel from the Hospice?

Hospice will be responsive to all concerns of Hospice patients and families. Hospice will encourage patients and family members to openly express their concerns, ask questions, and participate as fully as possible in their own care. When concerns take the form of complaints or grievances, Hospice personnel will respond as promptly as possible by addressing the issues and working toward a satisfactory solution to the problem. The Hospice goal is to provide comfort, compassionate care, and support to patients, their families, and significant others, enhancing the quality of their lives in positive and life-affirming ways.

Q: Will there be confidentiality regarding the patient's medical records and access to the patient's home?

"Hospice requires that no staff person, [contractual agent,] or volunteer will share information gained through their association with the Hospice with anyone not [specifically] authorized by Hospice to have access to such information." Each member of the Hospice staff, including volunteers, receives orientation to this effect and must sign a written "memorandum of understanding."

"Hospice guarantees that no staff or volunteer will enter the home of patients receiving Hospice services without the permission of the patient/family and/or primary caregiver, *and* the knowledge of the interdisciplinary team."

(See also "What about Confidentiality?" and "Memoranda of Understanding" in Chapter 10; and Appendix A, Figure 3, "Hospice Statement Prohibiting Redisclosure of Confidential Information.")

Reference

Hospice Operations Manual (Hempstead, NY: Long Island Foundation for Hospice Care and Research, Inc., 1990), p. 330.

Q: Is there ever a time when a patient will be discharged from the Hospice program?

Yes. The patient may request to be discharged. Or the condition of the patient stabilizes and the Hospice medical director or the patient's attending physician no longer consider the patient's condition to be terminal with a prognosis of six months or less to live. Or the patient/family move and no longer live in the service area of the Hospice. Or the primary caregiver is unable to be responsible for the patient and a new primary caregiver is not available, or there is no alternative "primary care support system" available. Living Hospice patients are not discharged because of inability to pay or because their insurance benefits expire. Discharge of patients is a rare or unusual circumstance.

Only 2.4 percent of patients entering a Hospice program were discharged. Thirty-four percent of discharges were due to a patient moving out of the area and/or another Hospice program; 19 percent were discharged to a hospital; 15 percent to a home health agency; and 21 percent were discharged for other reasons.

Reference

National Hospice Organization, "Hospice Fact Sheet" (Arlington, VA: Updated October 10, 1995).

Q: What happens when a patient dies at home? What does the family do?

Hospice guidelines are written for the staff and volunteers working with them to assist the families in understanding the steps that need to be taken after death has occurred in the home.

Certain procedures need to be followed at the time of death to meet the necessary legal requirements. Familiarity with these steps will help prevent unnecessary disruption and stress for the family at this emotionally charged time. The Hospice also wants to prevent needless involvement of police and emergency vehicles.

Hospice personnel in the home may prepare the deceased for release to the funeral home in accordance with the request of the family and the funeral director. The Hospice will contact any contracted agencies involved to cancel services and will arrange for equipment in the home to be picked up and returned to the appropriate agency.

The Hospice will notify the volunteers who have been involved with the patient and family of the patient's death.

It is expected that the persons involved with the Hospice patient and family will have reviewed these guidelines with the family prior to the death event. It is also expected that, whenever possible, supporting persons in the family's immediate network will be identified to be present at the death vigil or called at the time of death itself, if the family wishes. (Some families also may want a friend or pastoral care person to be there.)

Careful preparation prior to the time of death will help mobilize the resources of the family or neighborhood to be a supportive network. Hospice staff and volunteers may become involved at this time, if this seems to be needed and desired by the family and significant others.

3
CHILDREN

1. Is Hospice care appropriate for children with a terminal illness?

2. What about Hospice care for children who have a serious chronic illness?

3. Does the Hospice provide support services for the children who are family members of the terminally ill person?

Q: Is Hospice care appropriate for children with a terminal illness?

Yes. Hospice care is appropriate for terminally ill patients of all ages, children as well as adults. According to Children's Hospice International,

CHILDREN'S HOSPICE CARE supports the patient and family by providing professional, compassionate care. It involves an interdisciplinary team (physician, nurse, social worker, clergy, teachers, various therapists and specially trained volunteers) working together toward creating an atmosphere in which the patient and family can live life as fully as possible. It also involves bereavement support following the death....

The stress involved in caring for a seriously ill child is enormous, often resulting in an increase of disruptive behavior and psychosocial problems within the family. Hospice-type care can provide family members and significant others with appropriate support allowing the family members to grow stronger as individuals and as a family. It can turn a potentially devastating experience into a strengthening and bonding one.

Children's Hospice care allows parents to assume the role of primary caregiver and to have a voice in making decisions. The family is supported by an interdisciplinary team throughout the child's illness and through the first 13 months of bereavement.

Children's Hospice International "creates a world of Hospice support for children providing medical and technical assistance, research and education for these special children, their families and health care professionals." They can be contacted at: Children's Hospice International, 1850 M Street NW, Suite 900, Washington, DC 20036. (703) 684-0330, (800) 242-4453; FAX: (703) 684-0226.

Q: What about Hospice care for children who have a serious chronic illness?

According to Children's Hospice International, "Approximately 100,000 children die annually in the United States and about 1,000,000 children are seriously chronically ill. They and their families can benefit from Hospice-type care."

Usually Hospice program admission requires a medical prognosis of six months or less. The Hospice-type of care incorporates a support system and palliative care that are appropriate in caring for the children and their families, even prior to the end stages of chronic illness. Parents are encouraged to join support groups even during the chronic stage of the child's illness."

Q: Does the Hospice program provide support services for the children who are family members of the terminally ill person?

Yes, the needs of *all* family members, including children of any age, are addressed in the patient/family plan of care. (See also "What are some of the reactions one may expect from children when there is a death in the family?" "What is the role of children during the funeral?" "What do you tell children about death?"; and "How can children become involved when the patient is in the Hospice program?" in Chapter 11.)

The following publications can be helpful, as well as some of those listed in "Suggested Reading," Chapter 12.

Grollman, Earl A., *Explaining Death to Children* (Boston, MA: Beacon Press, 1967).

——, *Talking about Death: A Dialogue between Parent and Child* (Boston, MA: Beacon Press, 1976).

National Hospice Organization, *Journal: Special Pediatric Issue, Funded by Loewen Children's Foundation* (November 1995), 6(5).

Reynolds, Jeffrey L., writer and editor, *Reclaiming Lost Voices: Children Orphaned by HIV/AIDS in Suburbia* (Huntington Station, NY: Long Island Association for AIDS Care, Inc. [LIAAC], August 1995.)

References

Fact Sheet: Children's Hospice International, Inc. (CHI), (Washington, DC, 1992).

Pediatric AIDS Foundation (PAF), 1311 Colorado Avenue, Santa Monica, CA 90404 (1-800-488-5000) or (310) 395-9051.

4
AIDS

1. What is AIDS, and what is meant by "HIV Infection"?

2. How is HIV transmitted? What is meant by "casual" contact?

3. Why do people with AIDS find it difficult to accept Hospice care?

4. Does Hospice take away hope from persons with AIDS, the family, and significant others?

5. Will the AIDS patient, his family, and significant others be involved in the Hospice plan of care?

6. What are some other issues of concern for people with AIDS in regard to Hospice care?

7. What do Hospices do to educate and train their staff (including volunteers and contract staff) who work with HIV/AIDS patients?

8. Is the Hospice philosophy and care appropriate for people with AIDS, their families, and significant others? How can Hospice services help them?

9. Do most Hospices accept persons with AIDS into their programs? Are the Hospice admission criteria different for persons with various terminal conditions including HIV/AIDS?

10. What can a Hospice program offer persons with AIDS, their families, and significant others? What is "migration home" syndrome?

11. Is Hospice care different for people with HIV/AIDS than for people with cancer or other terminal conditions?

12. What are the bereavement implications of the "multiple losses" experienced by people living with HIV/AIDS, their families, and significant others?

13. How has the profile of persons living with AIDS changed over the past ten years?

14. What are AIDS Service Organizations (ASOs)? Can Hospices and ASOs collaborate to benefit the HIV/AIDS population?

15. Can you suggest some informative reading material about HIV/AIDS?

Q: What is AIDS, and what is meant by "HIV infection"?

Acquired Immunodeficiency Syndrome (AIDS) is a disease which impairs the body's immune system. This affects the body's ability to fight disease and leaves a person vulnerable to opportunistic infections; that is, infections that take advantage of the body's inability to resist disease.

It is important to distinguish between AIDS and the Human Immunodeficiency Virus (HIV) which causes AIDS. AIDS cannot be spread from one person to another, but HIV can be passed to other people through specific body fluids. A person with HIV infection can have no outward symptoms of illness. HIV infection refers to *all* people with the virus, while AIDS refers *only* to those in the final stage of HIV infection who have specific illnesses and conditions. In recognition of changing medical terminology, newly enacted statutes generally refer to HIV infection rather than AIDS (Rennert, 1989).

There are three distinct stages of HIV infection.

Asymptomatic HIV Infection

In this first stage, *asymptomatic HIV infection,* individuals do not have any visible symptoms to indicate illness. There can be quite a long incubation period, perhaps from eight to eleven years, before the onset of AIDS.

During the asymptomatic period, the infected *adult* remains healthy, gradually developing symptoms associated with HIV infection. The asymptomatic period is not as long for *infants* with congenital HIV infection; the majority of these infants will show HIV-related symptoms within the first year" (Rennert, 1989).

Symptomatic HIV Infection

Formerly referred to as "AIDS-related Complex (ARC)" " ... this category has passed out of use. T-cell counts are now used to distinguish when 'AIDS' begins (and T-cells may in the future cease to be a marker)" (Brenner, 1996). During this second stage, *symptomatic HIV infection,* there is the development of

. . .various clinical signs, including [opportunistic infections,] lympadenopathy (chronically swollen lymph nodes), weight loss, fever, diarrhea, thrush, general malaise, skin tumors, and other conditions. In *children*, there also may be unusual pulmonary infections which signal HIV; however, vague general symptoms are more likely, including failure to thrive, developmental delays or loss of previous developmental achievements, diarrhea, and recurrent bacterial infections (Rennert, 1989).

AIDS

The *third* phase, *AIDS*, is also a clinical diagnosis indicated by specific symptoms or diseases identified by the CDC [Centers for Disease Control], such as Kaposi's sarcoma and pneumocystis carinii pneumonia [PCP]. [HIV also is *neurotropic*, causing infections of the brain, spinal cord, and peripheral nervous system. These numerous neurological manifestations of AIDS lead increasingly to dependency and can include dementia, incontinence, paralysis, and blindness (*Executive Summary*, 1988).] Clinical studies suggest that as many as 50 to 70 percent of persons with AIDS will develop an organic mental disorder, including cognitive impairment, language disorder, movement disorders, psychosis, mood disorders, delirium and dementia. These mental disorders can begin either during the "symptomatic phase" or once a person has developed AIDS . . . included under the umbrella term "AIDS dementia complex." At the present time, AIDS is believed to be universally fatal.

[In *children*, the progression of HIV infection] is much more rapid than in adults; however, even in children HIV can have varying rates of progression. While a few infants die within months of being diagnosed, others can have a slow progression of health problems, while still other children have a long, relatively stable course. Some children with congenital HIV infection have reached eight years of age (Rennert, 1989).

In children and infants with congenital HIV infection, central nervous system involvement becomes one of the major clinical symptoms.

References

Brenner, Paul R., Exec. Dir., Jacob Perlow Hospice (New York: Private communication, May 1996).

Executive Summary: Plan for a Comprehensive Response to HIV Infection and Related Diseases in Nassau and Suffolk Counties (Plainview, NY: Nassau-Suffolk Health Systems Agency, November 1988).

Rennert, Sharon, et al. AIDS and Persons with Developmental Disabilities: The Legal Perspective (Washington, DC: American Bar Association, Commission on the Mentally Disabled, and Center on Children and the Law, 1989).

Q: How is HIV transmitted? What is meant by "casual" contact?

Significant Risk for HIV Infection

Only four routes of HIV transmission have been documented: (1) through unprotected sex (vaginal, oral or anal); (2) through transfusions or infusions of blood or blood products; (3) through sharing of intravenous needles [or other drug paraphernalia]; and (4) through congenital or perinatal transmission from [an infected] woman to her fetus or newborn child and, in a few cases, through breast-feeding. While blood has been identified as an agent for transmittal of HIV, transmission can only occur when infected blood comes into contact with an open wound [or skin with a dermatitis condition or with abraded areas]. Skin acts as a barrier to transmission; only if someone has an open wound, or receives an inoculation [or a blood transfusion] with HIV-infected blood, is there contact sufficient to risk transmission. Regardless of whether an individual has asymptomatic HIV infection or AIDS, once a person is infected he or she has the potential to transmit HIV to another person through one of the routes mentioned above. . . . [Also] health care workers risk exposure to HIV through accidental needle-sticks with blood from HIV-positive individuals. However, the rate of transmission as a result of such accidents has been less than one percent (Rennert, 1989).

Significant Risk Does Not Include

1. exposure to urine, feces, sputum, nasal secretions, saliva, sweat, tears, or vomitus that does not contain blood that is visible to the naked eye;
2. human bites where there is no direct blood to blood or blood to mucous membrane contact;
3. exposure of intact skin to blood or any other body substance;
4. occupational settings where individuals use scientifically accepted barrier techniques and preventive practices in circumstances which would otherwise pose a significant risk (N.Y.S. Pub. Health Law).

What Is Meant by "Casual" Contact?

HIV *cannot* be transmitted through "casual" contact, such as living in the same household, attending the same school, or working with a person who has HIV infection. Studies of the household contacts of persons with HIV infection found no evidence of transmission through nonsexual contacts. Researchers examined a variety of activities, including sharing household items (such as eating utensils, drinking glasses, toothbrushes, towels), sharing household facilities (such as beds, bath/showers, toilets), washing items used by HIV-positive individuals (such as dishes and clothes) and interacting with HIV-positive individuals (such as hugging, kissing, helping someone to bathe or eat) (Rennert, 1989).

References

New York State Public Health Law, Section 2786, Subchapter G of Title 10 (Health), Part 63.1 ("Definitions") and 63.9 ("Significant Risk"), January 1989.

Rennert, Sharon, et al. *AIDS and Persons with Developmental Disabilities: The Legal Perspective* (Washington, DC: published jointly by the American Bar Association, Commission on the Mentally Disabled, and the Center on Children and the Law, 1989).

Q: Why do people with AIDS find it difficult to accept Hospice care?

The person who has been living with the knowledge that he or she is infected with HIV that has developed into AIDS may find it difficult to seek Hospice care. Part of the reason is the need to acknowledge the far advanced nature of the disease by a person who usually is very young when the average life-span is now over 70 years. It is not a lack of awareness of the gravity of the situation, but rather that the will to live is strong and is expressed in hope for a remission or cure in order to have a meaningful life.

Treatment methods are becoming more sophisticated, and people with AIDS may be reluctant to enter into palliative care. To many persons with AIDS,

> Hospice care, with its focus on acceptance of [approaching] death and delivery of palliative and supportive care, [is] largely viewed . . . as inappropriate for AIDS patients. To [many of] these people, Hospice care represents an admission of failure—failure in that the disease becomes the acknowledged victor. It has been difficult to communicate the positive aspect [of Hospice] that supports their fighting spirit—the concept of the empowerment of the individual (Tehan, 1991).

This is pretty much the gay model and will be different for middle-class white gay men than people of color and other minorities, or women and children, or substance abusers, the poor, the homeless, etc. (See also "How Has the Profile of Persons Living with AIDS Changed Over the Past Ten Years?" in this chapter.)

> Many women with AIDS are poor and uneducated, managing on their own, infected by husbands, by boyfriends or by their partners as sex workers (prostitutes). Black and Hispanic women and children are significantly overrepresented in the population of women and children with HIV. These women tend to deny their own medical needs, often not seeking medical care until their symptoms are acute and they are very ill. Their own health takes a back seat to the other issues, problems or demands in their lives. It is concern for their children and the fear of losing them that drive many women to finally seek care. . . . The disclosure of HIV status is a paramount and highly charged

issue for women, especially if they have a child (or children) who is HIV positive (Brennan and Dennis, 1996).

Do they tell their family members, their partner(s), employer, the children's school? If so, they may risk rejection and alienation by family and friends, loss of their job, their living quarters, the children's rejection from school and by their peers. Acceptance of Hospice care is admitting they have the HIV/AIDS virus. Psychosocial intervention is greatly needed in planning for the care and custody, and the education of these children (barriers to permanency planning).

There is a disproportionately large representation of African Americans and Hispanics among persons living with HIV/AIDS, and an increasingly large number of Native Americans, including Eskimos. Many are heterosexual substance abusers. Their ethnic and cultural beliefs and behaviors, and world view, affect how they respond to an illness—and whether or not, or even when, they will accept the intervention of health-care providers (whom they may look upon as "outsiders"). Some may live in a ghetto-type of environment; others in rural or exurban areas, and elsewhere.

Perhaps they have had very little contact with the health care community and aren't aware of hospice; or . . . perhaps their focus is not on their health but on caring for their children, or, in some circumstances, obtaining drugs. . . . On a day-to-day basis, some people may find that substance addiction will be more pressing than their AIDS diagnosis. Active drug users often have painful, dramatic lives filled with tragedy. Sometimes the focus of care will shift away from the terminal illness and move toward providing shelter or food to patients and families (Grothe, ibid., 1996).

Former drug abusers may be resistant to accepting Hospice care because they "have concerns about taking narcotics to control pain while they are dying. This requires that we [Hospice caregivers] educate clients about the use of pain medication in symptom management and the differences between using narcotics to control pain versus to get high" (ibid.).

References

Brennan, David, and Dennis, Jeanne, "Psychosocial Issues of HIV/AIDS Care," in *Resource Manual for Providing Hospice Care to People Living with AIDS* (Arlington, VA: National Hospice Organization [NHO 1994-1995 AIDS Resource Committee], 1996), pp. 9-15.

Grothe, Thomas, "Clinical Issues of HIV/AIDS in Hospice," ibid., pp. 2-8.

Tehan, Claire, "The Cost of Caring for Patients with HIV Infection in Hospice," *The Hospice Journal*, (1991) 7(1/2):42.

Q: Does Hospice take away "hope" from persons with AIDS (PWAs), the family, and significant others?

Hospice, with its emphasis on changing, not eliminating hope, offers an alternative. It offers hope that the last weeks or months of life can be lived in dignity and relative comfort. In this age of self-empowerment, patients' rights and self-determination, people with a limited life expectancy have a right to choose how they want to live their last days. The mission of Hospice care is to meet the needs of the terminally ill patients who have decided to forego often futile and painful procedures and put aggressive symptom control first. Hospice care is not withdrawing care but changing [from cure to] care (Weber, 1992).

Reference

Weber, Jane, "Choosing Hospice Care: Things to Know," *PWA Coalition Newsline* (June 1992), (77):43.

Q: Will the AIDS patient, the family, and significant others be involved in the Hospice plan of care?

Yes. The Hospice staff acts in partnership with the physician, the patient, the family, and significant others to develop a plan of care that will put as much life as possible into the time that is left. The plan avoids treatment that would only prolong the patient's dying. *All* Hospice patients, including AIDS patients, are consulted and have a say not only in the overall objectives of their care but in the details.

Hospice care aims to give the patient control over his or her life and to remove obstacles toward that end. Home health aides [personal care aides, homemakers], visiting nurses, social workers, clergy, and volunteers regularly go to the patient's home to help them [patients] and their caregivers deal with the problems of the illness (Weber, 1992).

The Hospice interdisciplinary team, including the patient's physician, can play a significant supportive role in clarifying the issues in treatment decisions. In creating the individual plan of care, it would be helpful to consider and discuss the following.

- Regarding the intervention: What are the wishes and expectations of the patient, the family, and significant others?
- Regarding participation in making decisions: do the patient, family, and significant others have current, accurate information about the treatment alternatives for HIV/AIDS? What do they expect from the treatment?

The plan of care will indicate that the patient and any relatives or friends who are to be involved in the patient's care will be given written guidelines and be instructed on precautions that need to be taken in the home setting.

References

"Precautions to Be Taken in Caring for a Patient With AIDS," in *Hospice Operations Manual* (Hempstead, NY: Long Island Foundation for Hospice Care and Research, Inc., 1989), pp. 275-7.

Weber, Jane, "Choosing Hospice Care: Things to Know," *PWA Coalition Newsline* (June 1992), (77):43-4.

Q: What are some other issues of concern for people with AIDS in regard to Hospice care?

One outcome of the Amsterdam conference on AIDS in August 1992 was that AIDS is now considered a chronic long-term illness, with no cure at present—*and* with a terminal stage, but not necessarily in the terminal end-stage of the illness. This change is due to the ability to provide symptom control for AIDS patients, which has extended the life expectancy of the patient. With the diagnosis of AIDS, the prognosis is very difficult, since new treatments have become available. The patients also may want aggressive treatment until the end, in the hope that a remission or cure may occur.

Treatment protocols now call for beginning treatment of HIV infected individuals when they are asymptomatic, prior to the onset of the illness. This requires the monitoring of T-cell counts and starting patients on low doses of zidovudine (AZT) while they are still asymptomatic. Treatment ideally begins with the knowledge of serostatus (*Surveillance*, 1992).

Pneumocystis carinii pneumonia (PCP), one of the more common opportunistic infections associated with AIDS, has become less of a problem since the introduction of aerosolized pentamidine therapy and oral Bactrim. The other brand name is Septra. Also, the introduction of zidovudine (AZT) in low dosages while the patient is asymptomatic has increased the period of time between infection and illness, and hence between infection and AIDS (*Surveillance*, 1992).

Even so, *Wasting Syndrome* has become a significant symptom, according to Brenner (1996). While patients living with AIDS (PLWAs) *are* living longer because of these medications, "the body reaches a certain point where it just sort of gives out and the system collapses. There is a very rapid and progressive loss of weight—loss of body mass, muscular tone, and physical strength—and the body becomes profoundly weak. This [usually] happens suddenly, toward the end when death is imminent."

These patients might not meet the Medicare Hospice admission criteria or choose Hospice care; however, palliative, compassionate comfort care is always appropriate, from whatever source.

"Anticipatory grief," for the patient, family, and significant others, needs to be viewed with respect for culture and family support (or lack of support). (See also "What Is Meant by 'Anticipatory Grief'?" in Chapter 11.) Some families may find it difficult to accept the usual mode of transmission of the AIDS virus and the patient's lifestyle (which could be homosexual, bisexual, heterosexual, promiscuous, or involve intravenous drugs).

Other issues of concern, according to the Nassau-Suffolk Health Systems Agency, "include the insufficient and erratic reimbursement for the varying longevity of the illness, and the reluctance of patients to enter palliative [Hospice] care when treatment is available" (*Executive Summary*, 1988).

References

Brenner, Paul R., Exec. Dir., Jacob Perlow Hospice (New York: Private communication, May 1996).

Executive Summary: Plan for a Comprehensive Response to HIV Infection and Related Diseases in Nassau and Suffolk Counties (Plainview, NY: Nassau-Suffolk Health Systems Agency, 1988), pp. 10, 56, 57.

Surveillance of HIV infection, AIDS, and Related Illnesses in Nassau County (Plainview, NY: Nassau-Suffolk Health Systems Agency, 1992), pp. 22, 39.

Q: What do Hospices do to educate and train their staff (including volunteers and contract staff) who work with HIV/AIDS patients?

There is a dual objective in the education and training *all* Hospice programs provide for their staff (including volunteers and contract personnel) in their work involving people with HIV/AIDS (PWAs):

1. Since PWAs have a weakened immune system, adequate precautions must be taken to protect the patient as well as the caregiver from the transmission of contagions.
2. Providing an understanding of the HIV/AIDS syndrome will reduce any fear of contagion the caregiver(s) may have. Understanding the nuances of HIV infection will enable staff to provide quality Hospice care. In turn, they will educate the patient, family, and significant others regarding the reality and progression of the infection.

All new Hospice staff and volunteers (including board members, administration, and contract personnel) go through an orientation period that includes basic information about HIV/AIDS and the agency's policies and procedures. Written guidelines are given and updated when pertinent new information becomes available (*Hospice Operations Manual*, 1989).

Training includes guidelines for infection control and universal precautions to be taken for *all* Hospice patients. Inservices include instructions regarding confidentiality and disclosure of HIV-related information; the scope of available services; responsibilities and expectations of staff (and volunteers) in caring for persons with AIDS; and staff health issues. Also included are admission policies about AIDS—nondiscriminatory practices when admitting and caring for persons having or suspected of having HIV infection.

The NHO AIDS Task Force also recommends:

- Responsibility for AIDS education should be assigned. This might be a small group (multidisciplinary) with a lead person. An action plan for AIDS education should be developed to guide activities.
- Mechanisms to obtain up-to-date information and materials should be established.
- Staff and volunteers with direct patient contact should have formal and informal support services/interventions available to them.
- Hospice library resources should include current information about the epidemic and the care of patients with AIDS and should be available to all staff and volunteers.
- The AIDS education plan/activities should be closely integrated with the agency's quality assurance program in order to assure effective monitoring and evaluation.
- Periodic staff inservices for HIV/AIDS and mutual support sessions, plus stress-reduction programs, including bereavement support, are of great help in enabling Hospice caregivers to cope and continue to provide optimum compassionate care.

Members of the NHO 1994-1995 AIDS Resource Committee further recognize the need for (1) cultural competency education (for staff and volunteers, contractual support staff, families and significant others, as well as members of the larger community); and (2) the effects of *multiple losses* for PLWAs. (See also "How Has the Profile of Persons Living with AIDS Changed over the Past Ten Years?" and "What Are the Bereavement Implications of the 'Multiple Losses' Experienced by People Living with HIV/AIDS, Their Families, and Significant Others?" in this chapter.)

References

Kilburn, Linda H., "Palliative Care Guidelines for Persons with AIDS," in *Hospice Operations Manual* (Arlington, VA: National Hospice Organization, Inc. [NHO Task Force on AIDS], 1988), pp. 462-82.

National Hospice Organization (NHO), *Resource Manual for Providing Hospice Care to People Living with AIDS* (Arlington, VA: NHO 1994-1995 AIDS Resource Committee [1996]).

"Precautions to be Taken in Caring for a Patient with Acquired Immune Deficiency (AIDS)," in *Hospice Operations Manual* (Hempstead, NY: Long Island Foundation for Hospice Care and Research, Inc., 1989), pp. 275-7.

Q: Is the Hospice philosophy and care appropriate for people with AIDS, their families and significant others? How can Hospice services help them?

Yes, the Hospice philosophy and care provided can be appropriate for people with AIDS, their families, and significant others, when they meet the Hospice admission criteria.

The purpose of Hospice is to provide support and care for people in the final phase of a terminal disease so that they can live as fully and comfortably as possible. Hospice neither hastens nor postpones death. Hospice believes that through personalized services and a caring community, patients and families can attain the necessary preparation for a death that is satisfactory to them (Weber, 1992).

Since the patient and family are considered the "unit of care," the Hospice program also provides guidance and emotional support to all involved before and after the death of the loved one. Hospice philosophy is concerned with

- Helping patients to live with dignity, each moment of every day, for whatever time they have left
- Helping families to participate in the caregiving process, living to the fullest, each moment of each day

- Helping [the families and significant others] resolve their grief and rebuild their lives (*Brochure*, 1985).

The goal of the Hospice philosophy is to relieve and control pain and manage the symptoms of the illness, recognizing that the patient's condition is incurable. While this Hospice philosophy *is* appropriate for the care of the person with AIDS it may conflict with the goals of a number of AIDS patients, and perhaps their families or caregivers. At present,

> ... there is no cure for the HIV infection which causes AIDS ... [and] there is no treatment currently available to cure HIV disease. . . . The interventions currently available to treat the opportunistic infections and neoplasms associated with AIDS generally offer temporary symptomatic relief and often must be continued indefinitely to assure continued relief. Although difficult for many patients and their families or caregivers to accept, most available medications, even those for the minor infections associated with HIV disease, are truly palliative rather than curative (Martin, 1991).

Providing appropriate comprehensive and compassionate quality care for *all* terminal patients certainly includes persons with AIDS in the Hospice circle of care.

References

Brochure (Westbury, NY: Long Island Foundation for Hospice Care and Research, Inc., 1985).

Martin, Jeannee Parker, "Issues in the Current Treatment of Hospice Patients with HIV Disease," *The Hospice Journal* (1991), 7(1/2):31-40.

Weber, Jane, "Choosing Hospice Care: Things to Know," *PWA Coalition Newsline* (June 1992), (77):43-4.

Q: Do most Hospices accept persons with AIDS into their programs? Are the Hospice admission criteria different for persons with various terminal conditions including HIV/AIDS?

More and more Hospices are accepting persons with AIDS into their programs, recognizing that caring for persons with AIDS presents a challenge. It involves (among other things) dealing with different types of stress; being creative in providing a primary care system for those who do not have a primary caregiver or a safe home environment; learning new clinical skills; and seeking out the financial resources necessary for the provision of comprehensive quality care.

The basic admission criteria are the same for *all* Hospice patients (Weber, 1992):

- Patient diagnosed as having advanced disease with a limited life expectancy
- Patient under the care of a licensed physician [as well as the Hospice physician] agree that Hospice care is appropriate
- Patient resides in geographical area that the Hospice serves
- Patient and caregiver consent to Hospice services. [This means they have chosen palliative care and no longer seek a cure for the disease.]
- Primary care person in the home is preferred, or a primary care system available. ["Some Hospices require this, some do not, and those programs most open to AIDS patients do not. Many persons with AIDS in urban areas live alone and have no family caregivers"] (Brenner, 1996).
- Race, creed, color, religion, national origin, sex, sexual orientation, disability, disease, age, marital status, or ability to pay does not determine a patient's eligibility for Hospice care.

The growing awareness and understanding of the nature of HIV infection and the complexity of the issues involved in caring for persons with AIDS have led to the increasing realization that the Hospice program of palliative care can benefit people with HIV/AIDS *and* their families.

Hospice programs are trying to relax their admission criteria to ensure that their array and intensity of services are available to [persons with AIDS and their families]. For the patient with advanced diseases, Hospice offers a holistic approach to reduce pain, and [provides] services to support the patient at home for as long as possible.

Hospice can provide understanding and relief for caregivers, friends, family, and volunteers who have often had too many losses. To die and to LIVE in dignity is very much in the hearts and minds of Hospice providers (Weber, 1992).

A major issue of concern in the Hospice admission process for persons with AIDS involves medical protocol and interventions. Are the prescribed treatments palliative or curative? ("With AIDS, no treatment is 'curative.' The issue is more in the use of life-extending treatments" [Brenner, 1996].) What is the goal of any intravenous therapy? As an example, many discussions concern whether total parenteral intervention (TPN) is appropriate for a Hospice patient. Although it is most likely that Hospice clinicians would *not* recommend using TPN for terminally ill patients, they might reconsider using this therapy if the goal is to promote the emotional and physical well-being of both the family and the patient. Even so, "TPN or hydration should not be considered for long term maintenance in any terminally ill patient. The risks and costs far outweigh the benefits" (Martin, 1991).

According to Claire Tehan, with over twenty years in the Hospice movement:

> . . . with continually emerging treatments . . . there is little agreement about what constitutes curative and what constitutes palliative care. What is aggressive treatment for AIDS? Is AZT, relieving symptoms and extending life for a short time, palliative? Should aerosol pentamidine isothionate and DHPG [long term ganciclovir] infusion, prophylactic drugs that prevent pneumonia and CMV [cytomegalovirus] retinitis respectively, be considered palliative or curative? [Is their use appropriate when the patient has only a short time to live?] There is as yet no accepted standard. Each Hospice decides what is within the scope of its particular program. Physicians and persons with AIDS view this uncertainty as a limitation of their options (Tehan, 1991).

The National Hospice Organization (NHO) 1994-1995 AIDS Resource Committee states:

People with HIV disease are often receiving what [some] hospices might perceive as curative or aggressive treatments. However, we do not believe there are interventions, drugs or treatments which can be universally viewed as inappropriate in the service of hospice care. . . . It is not the intervention but the goal that should be considered when evaluating a treatment's appropriateness in hospice. Therefore, we believe there can be times when IV [intravenous] medication, hydration, prophylaxis, antibiotics, suppressive therapies and even radiation and chemotherapy can be appropriate to the hospice plan of care. If the goal of treatment is to control symptoms, and that treatment is the soundest clinical intervention to achieve these results, then such treatments should be part of hospice" (National Hospice Organization, 1996, p. 3).

The acceptance of *any* patient into the Hospice program, regardless of the nature of the terminal illness, depends upon (1) the scope and resources available to the individual Hospice, (2) whether a patient meets the admission criteria, and (3) whether the Hospice program can meet the staffing requirements and financial costs of providing the greater intensity and level of care (psychosocial and spiritual, as well as physical) usually required for AIDS patients.

References

Brenner, Paul R., Exec. Dir., Jacob Perlow Hospice (New York, Personal communication, May 1996).

Martin, Jeannee Parker, "Issues in the Current Treatment of Hospice Patients with HIV Disease," *The Hospice Journal* (1991), 7(1/2):31-40.

Miller, Robert J., "Some Notes on the Impact of Treating AIDS Patients in Hospices," *The Hospice Journal* (1991), 7(1/2):1-12.

National Hospice Organization (NHO), *Resource Manual for Providing Hospice Care to People Living with AIDS* (Arlington, VA: NHO 1994-1995 AIDS Resource Committee [1996]), p. 3.

Tehan, Claire, "The Cost of Caring for Patients With HIV Infection in Hospices," *The Hospice Journal* (1991), 7(1/2):41-59.

Weber, Jane, "Choosing Hospice Care: Things to Know." *PWA Coalition Newsline* (June 1992), (77):43-4.

Q: What can a Hospice program offer persons with AIDS, their families, and significant others? What is "migration home" syndrome?

Paul Wright, Boston AIDS activist, states:

I think it's important to think of Hospice as an invitation to the patient. It is an opportunity to consider alternatives and to collaborate in his or her own life's journey, even if that journey is close to the end. Hospice offers an opportunity to demonstrate what it means to celebrate life in a very different way—an opportunity for people to reflect and to gather bits and pieces of their lives (Beresford, 1989).

A Hospice program can offer persons with AIDS, their families, and significant others the following services (Weber, 1992):

- Regularly scheduled home visits by the Hospice team members to evaluate the patient's condition and to supervise care
- Instructions to the caregiver(s) on management of the physical and emotional symptoms such as pain, anxiety, confusion, or poor appetite
- Assistance with the personal care of the patient (such as bathing, feeding, linen changes)
- Companionship for the patient if the family has to be out of the home for a short period of time
- Transportation, supplies, equipment, and medication
- 24-hour on-call availability
- Emotional support and counseling for both the patient and caregivers
- Spiritual care that is sensitive to the needs of all faiths [and lifestyles]
- Occupational, physical, speech, and music therapies and nutritional counseling
- Short term hospitalization and respite care for problems that cannot be managed at home

The Hospice program also can offer further education, guidance, and assistance by qualified staff in creating a safe home environment, which may also include reaching out to other "home environments," by coordinating with (1) a residence or SRO (single room occupancy hotel); (2) a substance abuse program; and/or (3) managing daily care needs, etc., ". . . to provide adequate protection from the transmission of contagens to *both* the patient and the caregiver [including the family and significant others, as well as staff and volunteers in other programs]."

"The primary nurse will make a home visit prior to giving any care, to ensure [that universal precautions are followed and] the home is set up and equipped appropriately for the patient's condition at the time of admission" ("Precautions," 1989).

For persons with AIDS who enter the Hospice program without a full-time primary care person or have only a part-time caregiver available *or* who live alone *or* in an unsafe environment *or* whose family and friends *do* want to help but are not able to *or* choose not to do so for a variety of reasons, some Hospice programs can offer assistance in creating cooperative arrangements with other community programs and organizations. (See also "Why Is Having a Primary Caregiver So Important to the Patient in a Hospice Program?" in Chapter 2 and "What Are AIDS Service Organizations (ASOs)? Can Hospices and ASOs Collaborate to Benefit the HIV/AIDS Population?" in this chapter.)

This may include participation in an adult day care program, with transportation and therapeutic activities providing the opportunity to socialize with others. (See also "What Is Hospice Day Care?" in Chapter 9.)

With the necessary cooperation of the patient, a primary care support system could be arranged by appropriate Hospice staff for the patient's shelter, safety, and adequate level and quality of care.

"In addition, it is recommended that prior to admission to Hospice or as soon as possible thereafter, the [person with AIDS] be strongly encouraged to make arrangements for durable power of attorney for both financial and for health care decisions. The designated person(s) may or may not be the primary care person(s)" (Kilburn, 1988). (See also "How Can the Patient and Family Be Assured Their Wishes Will Be Made Known to the Hospice Team ['Advance Directives']?" in Chapter 6.)

"Migration Home" Syndrome

Hospice programs can provide invaluable support addressing complex issues brought about by the *migration home syndrome*—the issue of adult children returning home ". . . to be cared for in their last days by their family of origin." As young people tend to do, many left home (whether urban, suburban, or rural) ". . . to find jobs, education and greater professional and personal opportunity. Now, with no job and little resources . . ." and faced with HIV/AIDS, these adult children have left behind their social support, experiencing the loss of their partners, peers, and families of choice (many of whom may have died). Facing the reality of the trajectory of their HIV/AIDS disease, they now also may be confronted by a family and community "attitude" regarding homophobia, their lifestyles, ignorance about HIV/AIDS disease and its progression, the possible ". . . complicating factors of illegal drug use, prostitution, antisocial behavior and/or dementia. Families are sometimes coping with thoughts and feelings about the lifestyle of the HIV-positive family member at the same time they are dealing with the reality of impending death [of a young person]. Caring for these patients [and their families] can challenge even the most skilled clinician" (Brown and Mawn, 1996), and involve all the members of the interdisciplinary team, working closely together in creating and implementing the patient/family plan of care.

References

Beresford, Larry, "The Challenge of AIDS," *California Hospice Report* (Summer/Fall 1989), 1(3):1-16.

Brown, Gretchen, and Mawn, David, "Rural Issues," in *Resource Manual for Providing Hospice Care to People Living with AIDS* (Arlington, VA: National Hospice Organization [NHO 1994-1995 AIDS Resource Committee], 1996), pp. 35-6.

Kilburn, Linda H., "Palliative Care Guidelines for Persons with AIDS," in *Hospice Operations Manual* (Arlington, VA: National Hospice Organization, [NHO Task Force on AIDS], 1988), pp. 462-82.

"Precautions to Be Taken in Caring for a Patient with AIDS," in *Hospice Operations Manual* (Hempstead, NY: Long Island Foundation for Hospice Care and Research, Inc., 1989), pp. 275-7.

Weber, Jane, "Choosing Hospice Care: Things to Know," *PWA Coalition Newsline* (June 1992), (77):43-4.

Q: Is Hospice care different for people with HIV/AIDS than for people with cancer or other terminal conditions?

The focus of Hospice care is the same for *all* patients, whatever the nature of the physical condition and the terminal illness.

- To keep the patients free from pain, as well as free from the fear of anticipatory pain, in relation to their illness
- To neither shorten life nor prolong the dying process, with death considered to be a natural part of life
- To consider the ill person and family together as a whole, with services offered to both, and to help them to live a quality life with dignity, for whatever time is left—by providing a coordinated interdisciplinary program of compassionate care and supportive services in a life-affirming environment
- To provide extended care to support grieving family members and significant others, before and during bereavement, for at least one year after the death
- To be available to patients and families, 24 hours a day, 7 days a week, and to encourage patients, families, and significant others to take an active role in the planning and care provided (*Brochure*, 1985).

According to the National Hospice Organization Task Force on AIDS, "There are major differences in the specifics of care [for persons with AIDS]—differences in medical management, psychosocial problems, and in some instances, the nature of the spiritual support required" (Kilburn, 1988). Robert Miller states:

That AIDS patients and their families require more intensive levels of support services and that the patients, themselves, are more difficult to treat clinically than are traditional hospice patients is well known. These patients are relatively young. Many present pain control difficulty because of a long-standing history of drug abuse. More than half of them have severe and persistent diarrheas. Others have progressive dementia and blindness. Additionally there are the psychosocial problems of [culture and] life style issues, and lack of traditional, and in some cases "alternative" family support (Librach, 1987). Some of these patients are totally abandoned [indigent and homeless]. They suffer social stigmatization, and because of life style issues, have an increased need for confidentiality and privacy (Gilmore, 1987).

"More recently, recognition of the sudden onset of *wasting syndrome* requires intensive supervision and care as the AIDS patient becomes profoundly weak" (Brenner, 1996).

At different times during their terminal stage of illness, persons with AIDS may require more kinds and more expensive medications (which might *traditionally* be considered invasive and aggressive, "curative" therapy for other patients who do not have AIDS). These treatments for opportunistic infections and neoplasms, although they may offer only temporary relief in symptom control, really are palliative, not curative. Since there is presently no known cure for the HIV virus, most available medications are given to control pain, manage the infections and symptoms, and slow down the progress of the illness.

Because the trajectory of the illness AIDS is so different from other terminal illnesses, the interface between curative and palliative treatment is more blurred than Hospices are accustomed to (e.g., AIDS patients who are experiencing the first or second bout of pneumocystis carinii pneumonia are routinely treated with antibiotics; intravenous or rehydration therapy, secondary to severe diarrhea, is often initiated as the treatment of choice) (Kilburn, 1988).

The NHO Task Force on AIDS suggests that Hospices consider the following questions when making decisions regarding medical interventions.

- Is there sound medical rationale for instituting palliative treatment?
- Are there any alternatives which are less invasive or noninvasive which would effectively relieve discomfort or distressing symptoms?
- Are the potential benefits of therapy greater than the possible risks?
- Does the therapy require a prolonged inpatient stay?

- If the patient is hospitalized, what is the home care potential? Is it feasible to manage the patient at home during or following treatment?
- What are the resources (emotional, financial) of the patient and family?
- What can the Hospice program offer in terms of technical expertise and capability regarding these treatments?
- What are the financial resources of the Hospice with regard to these treatments?

Persons with AIDS may at times require more frequent nursing visits, more nutritional and dietary guidance, more care from home health and personal care aides, and homemaker services. The complexity of their psychosocial, spiritual, emotional, and financial needs will require a greater intensity and level of care due to their age and the perceived stigma of the diagnosis; increasing physical, financial, and social dependency; feelings of alienation, rejection, low self-esteem, and isolation; feelings of helplessness and lack of control over the HIV infection, their lives, and what is happening to their bodies. There may be problems with family intervention (or lack of it), including:

- Identification and resolution of issues such as open/closed communication; secrets regarding lifestyles, diagnosis, conflicts between family of origin and lover/companion
- Fear of contagion
- Fear of mortality among friends
- Family's fear of stigma and social isolation
- Awareness of possible substance abuse by other family members
- Need for education of family members re: transmission of disease [including universal precautions in the home] and safe sex; testing; substance abuse (Kilburn, 1988).

Most Hospice programs find it very helpful to network and tap into other support systems and community resources. There is a need "for Hospice staff to become actively involved in the HIV service network" (Tehan, 1991). (See also "What Are AIDS Service Organizations [ASOs]? Can Hospices and ASOs Collaborate to Benefit the HIV/AIDS Population?" in this chapter.) Because of the scope and financial costs of the services involved, the NHO Task Force on AIDS considers:

- Essential [the development of] relationships with multiple community resources and work toward a coordinated system of care within the gay community or with substance abuse treatment programs or health departments
- Increased need for crisis intervention with regard to patient's basic needs of housing, food, transportation, financial resources, legal problems
- Coordinate/refer persons with AIDS and their families to appropriate support groups in the community (e.g., foster parents support group, mothers of persons with AIDS, gay community) (Kilburn, 1988).

The bereavement component of the Hospice program may require different specific interventions regarding the biological family, the lover/companion of the person with AIDS, and those families with a history of substance abuse. Reverend William Doubleday stresses "the importance of sensitive funerals and memorial services and the need for serious bereavement follow-up." (See also "What Are the Bereavement Implications of the 'Multiple Losses' Experienced by People Living with HIV/AIDS, Their Families, and Significant Others?" in this chapter.)

Many persons with AIDS may not have a primary careperson or a primary care system available or in place when applying for Hospice admission. Hospice staff may need to

explore cooperative arrangements with other community organizations and programs in order to meet the multiple needs of persons with AIDS. [In providing spiritual support, consider that] many persons with AIDS are alienated from formal religion and have no church affiliation. Yet, as one faces death, the patient inevitably confronts the issues of self-identity, the meaning of life, and individual destiny. In ministering to the person with AIDS, the pastoral caregiver may have to break through the patient's negative images of God as a harsh judge, or the perception that spirituality is the special preserve of religious persons.

It is important that the Hospice team, particularly the pastoral caregiver, stress spirituality and not religious practice. It may be necessary for the team to explore non-traditional means to provide relevant spiritual support to persons with AIDS. It is essential that the pastoral caregiver respect the conscience and integrity of each person with AIDS. Clearly, it is not the pastoral caregiver's role to reinforce or repudiate a person's lifestyle, but simply to offer non-judgmental aid to the person with AIDS and his or her significant others. The central role of pastoral care is to provide genuine empathy and a transcendent perspective for the harsh reality of dying young (Kilburn, 1988).

Bereavement care in rural communities can be affected by their relative isolation, and can present additional challenges. Hospice staff frequently face issues which affect care, such as ignorance about the disease, judgmental attitudes (including homophobia, substance abuse, and promiscuity). There are always concerns about confidentiality for both the patient and the family, regardless of where they live, but the fear of revealing the AIDS diagnosis in small rural communities can be more intense due to attitude, religion, and psychosocial issues.

In rural areas confidentiality is supplanted for some families with the demand for secrecy. The secrecy issue means that referrals may be late because patients and families know hospice staff will likely know them. Volunteers, although badly needed, are often not accepted by the patient and/or family because of the focus on secrecy. The patient often is unable to honestly acknowledge his/her illness with friends and family members at a time when honesty in closure is critical; and family members' grief is often complicated because they cannot share the totality of their grief. Indeed, they are often constrained in the therapeutic "telling of their story" for fear a detail might reveal the true disease... [This is compounded by] few support groups exist in rural areas because the numbers of people who might use the group are scarce and the anonymity of the city is lacking" (Brown and Mawn, 1996).

References

Brochure (Westbury, NY: Long Island Foundation for Hospice Care and Research, Inc., 1985).

Brown, Gretchen, and Mawn, David, "Rural Issues," in *Resource Manual for Providing Hospice Care to People Living with AIDS* (Arlington, VA: National Hospice Organization [NHO 1994-1995 AIDS Resource Committee], 1996), pp. 32-8.

Doubleday, Rev. William A., "AIDS: Giving Direct, Helpful Care. Part II: Spiritual and Psychosocial Supports" *Trinity News* (March 1986), pp. 12-13.

Executive Summary: Plan for a Comprehensive Response to HIV Infection and Related Diseases in Nassau and Suffolk Counties (Plainview, NY: Nassau-Suffolk Health Systems Agency, Inc., 1988), pp. 10, 16, 53-7, 61-3.

Gilmore, N., "AIDS Palliative Care: The Courage to Care," *Journal of Palliative Care* (1987), 3(2):33-8.

Kilburn, Linda H., "Palliative Care Guidelines for Persons With AIDS," *Hospice Operations Manual* (Arlington, VA: National Hospice Organization, Inc. [NHO Task Force on AIDS], 1988), pp. 462-82.

Librach, S. L., "Acquired Immunodeficiency Syndrome: The Challenge for Palliative Care," *Journal of Palliative Care* (1987), 3(2):31-3.

Miller, Robert J., "Some Notes on the Impact of Treating AIDS Patients in Hospices," *The Hospice Journal* (1991), 7(1/2):1-12.

Tehan, Claire, "The Cost of Caring for Patients with HIV Infection in Hospice," *The Hospice Journal* (1991), 7(1/2):41-59.

Worden, William J., "Grieving a Loss From AIDS," *The Hospice Journal* (1991), 7(1/2):143-50.

Q: What are the bereavement implications of the "multiple losses" experienced by people living with HIV/AIDS, their families, and significant others?

In the Hospice bereavement program (including the "anticipatory grief" component), those being served are usually dealing with the death of one person at that particular time, and the approach to their bereavement care is based on this. (See Chapter 11 on Bereavement.) Dealing with one significant loss at a time enables them to become involved in the primary therapeutic intervention . . . to "normalize" the experience of loss and grief in order to prevent a "pathologizing" of the symptoms of the bereaved. While bereavement may be complicated or influenced by other mental health conditions, bereavement in and of itself is a normal aspect of the human experience . . . The process the bereaved are working through is most often assisted by helping them to externalize their feelings and emotions rather than holding them in. Expressing the feeling of loss will help the bereaved to integrate the loss into their ongoing experience and enable their lives to move forward. . . . Complications . . . involve losses which occur as a result of catastrophe, such as accidents, acts of violence, acts of nature or suicide, and losses which occur out of the sequence of "normal" life, such as the death of minor dependent children, or the loss of a parent [or sibling] by a young child.

As AIDS has changed every aspect of health care it has touched, it is also challenging the way bereavement care is understood, practiced and provided through hospices, AIDS Service Organizations and other community bereavement programs (Brenner, 1996).

The numbers of "multiple losses" to HIV/AIDS—deaths which have decimated their community (gays, lesbians, substance abusers, and their significant others)—have affected their very identity on functional, vocational, psychological, and spiritual levels. They have seen their partners and families of choice, their friends, peers and associates, experience the vicissitudes of the "roller coaster" effects of the disease—and died.

Because "many people living with HIV/AIDS have experienced [these] multiple losses to HIV [they] may be experiencing bereavement overload. They are aware of the potential course of the illness. This can create great stress on a patient, the family, and significant others as they are facing hospice care. Given this information, PLWAs may require more patience and support in trusting the goals of hospice care" (Brennan and Dennis, 1996). (See also "What Is Meant by 'Anticipatory Grief'?" in Chapter 11.)

"The perverse nature of the disease often finds these dying individuals able to be up and around and able to participate in community life, but without a community. The extraordinary grief and loss of a person who is losing his/her life through a disease characterized by myriad losses is intensified by the loss of home and friends and other social supports" (Brown and Mawn, 1996).

Persons living with HIV/AIDS may be particularly vulnerable when circumstances indicate they need to change their locale and they chose to "come home," to die in the care of their family of origin. (See *Migration Home Syndrome* in this chapter.)

Paul Brenner characterizes multiple losses ("Bereavement: Structuring Response to Losses Due to AIDS," 1996):

- Unlike the ability to "normalize" the feelings of loss and grief of many bereaved persons who are working through the loss of one significant person in their lives at a time, losses of the scope that are being experienced by members of the gay and lesbian community [and heterosexual intravenous drug abusers] cannot be normalized. *Catastrophic multiple losses overwhelm survivors* [my emphasis] creating layers which fuse together in an undifferentiated mass of pain, anger, mourning, sadness, numbness, disorder, confusion, and chaos, which is always threatening to break through and beyond the boundaries of containment. The threat that is constant is that one will be overwhelmed and rendered immobile and nonfunctional. The task of survivors of this kind of loss is to find ways to contain the loss so that they can continue to function in some way in life, in roles, in relationships.

- Uniquely affected are staff members of ASOs and hospice programs with a large AIDS census who are also gay and who may be HIV positive as well. Containing their losses in order to maintain job function cannot only affect the ability of staff to do their own work, but may also affect the way they relate to patients who have AIDS. The slogan, "Stay Alive For The Cure," may have a shadow side to it, as people with advanced AIDS may feel pressure to continue to fight at any cost when they are actually ready to let go, merely to give hope and courage to those who are living in earlier stages of the disease.

- Finally, even for members of families of origin who may *not* have experienced multiple losses due to AIDS, their bereavement is complicated by the framing of their loss within the stigma of homosexuality, addiction, or both, the loss of their expectations of their son fulfilling the heterosexual continuation of the family, their belief that they may have caused their son's homosexuality due to parenting errors or mistakes, or even that this may be divine punishment for some terrible sin they committed. Guilt and shame can be very crippling to the healing process for families, especially parents.

Prior to the patient's death, the anticipatory grief part of the program needs to include AIDS-specific issues in the risk assessment of survivors, including identification of ASOs and other appropriate materials and resources. In recognizing the importance of cultural competency, Hospice programs can network with and make referrals to those ASOs that may offer special support groups and counseling for persons living with HIV/AIDS, including Latinos, African Americans, Asians, Native Americans, women, children, and adolescents, and non-gays.

After the death of the patient, bereavement care is provided in most Hospice programs for 12 or 13 months. However, this time-frame may not be adequate to help those affected by HIV/AIDS. The usual services for family members and significant others may include staff/volunteer attendance at the wake and/or funeral, home visits during the official mourning period, as well as follow-up phone, calls, condolence letters and other correspondence, educational events, group and individual support groups and counseling, and when indicated, referrals to other community and professional services.

In dealing with losses due to HIV/AIDS, the usual 12- to 13-month Hospice bereavement period may *not* be appropriate.

The degree to which issues of sexuality, drug use, guilt, shame, religious ideation and the stigma of AIDS itself are enmeshed into the loss of a family member will not only complicate the grief issues and process, but will add to the time involved in finding some kind of satisfactory resolution. . . . Those who are multiply bereaved, especially members of the gay and lesbian community, may not be able to see any kind of resolution as being possible as long as the holocaust of deaths continues. Therefore, the time assumptions providers work within may need to focus more upon assuming a role without the assumption they will be able to complete the process with and for the bereaved. This may be an area in which local ASOs, gay and lesbian services organizations, community bereavement programs, and hospices could come together for collaboration and coordination (Brenner, 1996).

Brenner also suggests

... Rather than assuming it is always best to express the grief, thereby, threatening "flooding," it may be best to help individuals find ways to contain the loss, maintain function, and develop the inner resources to confront the pain over a much longer period of time ... [and incorporating] a holistic approach stressing rest, diet, diet supplements, support of the immune system, elimination of all unnecessary stress, controlling alcohol and drug use for numbing purposes, and use of meditation, stress reduction techniques, acupuncture, [therapeutic touch], and other related therapies (ibid).

References

Brennan, David, and Dennis, Jeanne, "Psychosocial Issues of HIV/AIDS Care," in *Resource Manual for Providing Hospice Care to People Living with AIDS* (Arlington, VA: National Hospice Organization [NHO 1994-1995 AIDS Resource Committee], 1966), p. 10.

Brenner, Paul R., "Bereavement: Structuring Response to Losses Due to AIDS," ibid., pp. 19-26.

Brown, Gretchen, and Mawn, David, "Rural Issues," ibid., p. 35.

Q: How has the profile of persons living with AIDS changed over the past ten years?

The profile of persons living with AIDS (PLWAs) has changed dramatically over the past ten years. In the early 1980s, AIDS patients were primarily young, white, middle-class gay men, followed by male intravenous drug abusers, and a few people (of both sexes) infected by blood transfusions during surgical procedures. According to a Federal Centers for Disease Control (CDC) report published in 1995, this early profile has changed dramatically.[1] Today, it encompasses people with diverse cultural backgrounds, women and children, the poor, the homeless, and a large percentage with substance abuse problems.

Women became the fastest growing population among AIDS cases. In 1985, 7 percent of AIDS cases were women; in 1994, it more than doubled, to 18 percent.[2] In 1994, the 14,081 cases reported among women for that year alone was almost 25 percent of the 58,448 female cases diagnosed since the beginning of the epidemic, in 1981.[3] Forty-one percent of women diagnosed in 1994 were infected through intravenous drug use; 38 percent through heterosexual contact with an infected partner;[4] and 19 percent reported they had no identifiable risk (although it was believed that most of those cases could be attributed to heterosexual transmission).[5]

The mode of transmission has changed.

Heterosexual transmission represents the largest proportionate increase in total AIDS cases in recent years. Transmission related to drug use has surpassed transmission related to men having sex with men. . . . Growing numbers of teenagers are infected with HIV. A discussion of adolescent sexual activity is taboo in many families, schools and churches. Teenagers engage in high risk sexual behavior; 11-13 year-olds are having unprotected sex. Drug and alcohol use are linked to high-risk sex because of lowered inhibitions under the influence of these substances. . . . Teenagers are not young adults and do not respond to the same messages or rationales that adults do. They may be aware of the consequences of high-risk behavior but take no precaution. Teenagers are egocentric, oriented to [the] present not future, have a vague sense of personal vulnerability and are heavily influenced by peers (Brennan and Dennis, 1996).

African Americans and Hispanics are statistically over-represented among persons living with AIDS (PLWAs). Increasing numbers of Native Americans, including Eskimos, have become infected with HIV/AIDS. The current rates of increase are greatest for women and children of color. More than 75 percent of the 1994 AIDS diagnoses were among African Americans and Hispanics.[6] Rates for Hispanic women were 7 times those of white women, while rates for women of color were 16 times higher than for those of white women.[7]

The great majority of PLWAs are in their late teens through the 40s; and then there are the children. According to the Long Island Association for AIDS Care (1995),

> Eighty-one percent of the women diagnosed through 1994 were between the ages of 20 and 49.[8] These are prime child-bearing years and the CDC's Survey in Childbearing Women reveals that an estimated 7,000 HIV-infected U.S. women delivered infants in 1993.[9] Assuming a perinatal transmission rate of 15 to 30 percent, approximately 1,000 to 2,000 infants were perinatally infected with HIV during 1993.[10] But again, these startling numbers are only the tip of the iceberg; thousands of other uninfected children and young adults will be forced to say good-bye to one or both parents before they see their eighteenth birthdays (Reynolds, 1995).

The report continues

> Though cancer remains the top killer, AIDS now steals more mothers from their children than most other major causes of death including motor vehicle accidents. By the end of this year [1995], an estimated 24,600 children, 21,000 adolescents and 35,100 young adults in the United States will be orphaned by the AIDS epidemic.[11] In the next five years, the numbers are projected to grow by leaps and bounds as between 72,000 and 125,000 American children lose their mothers.[12] An additional 60,000 young adults over the age of eighteen will see their moms die because of AIDS.[13]

These profile changes in PLWAs stress the importance of education and training in *cultural competency,* not only for Hospice staff and volunteers, but for all who are involved. "It is important to acknowledge that within each culture vast differences exist among individuals based upon age, gender, social class, number of generations in the United States, sexual orientation, level of education, and acculturation" (Brennan and Dennis, 1996).

So important has this become today, that the American Counseling Association has created a new division, the *Association for Multicultural Counseling and Development.*[14]

Issues of culture, ethnicity, race, age, gender and sexual orientation have assumed paramount importance as a result of population shifts and the growing national awareness of differences. ... There is a growing need [for all professional counselors and caregivers] to be aware of and sensistive to the many racial and ethnic groups, cultures, languages, values and belief systems of the publics we serve (Private communication, 1996).

References

Brennan, David, and Dennis, Jeanne, "Psychosocial Issues of HIV/AIDs Care," in *Resource Manual for Providing Hospice Care to People Living with AIDS* (Arlington, VA: National Hospice Organization [NHO 1994-1995 AIDS Resource Committee], 1996), pp. 9-15.

Reynolds, Jeffrey L., writer and editor, *Reclaiming Lost Voices: Children Orphaned by HIV/AIDS in Suburbia* (Huntington Station, NY: Long Island Association for AIDS Care, Inc. [LIAAC], August, 1995), pp. 20-1, 25-6.

Footnotes

1. Centers for Disease Control (CDC), "Update: Acquired Immunodeficiency Syndrome—United States, 1994," in *Morbidity and Mortality Weekly Report* (1995), 44:64-7.

2. Ibid.

3. Centers for Disease Control, *Facts About Women and HIV/AIDS,* February 13, 1995.

4. Centers for Disease Control, *HIV/AIDS Surveillance Report,* 1994 Year-End Report (January 1995), p. 5.

5. Ibid.

6. Ibid., p. 16.

7. Ibid.

8. Ibid.

9. Centers for Disease Control, "Update: AIDS Among Women—United States, 1994," in *Morbidity and Mortality Weekly Report* (1995), 44:n.p.

10. Gwinn, M., Pappaioanou, M., George, J.R., et al., "Prevalence of HIV Infection in Childbearing Women in the United States," *JAMA* (1994), 265:1704-8.

11. Michaels, D., and Levine, C., "Estimates of the Number of Youth Orphaned by AIDS in the United States," *JAMA* (1992), 268:3456-61.

12. Ibid.

13. Ibid.

14. Association for Multicultural Counseling and Development (Division of American Counseling Association), 5999 Stevenson Avenue, Alexandria, VA 22304-3300; (703) 823-9800 (Private communication, 1996).

Q: What are AIDS Service Organizations (ASOs)? Can Hospices and ASOs collaborate to benefit the HIV/AIDS population?

AIDS Service Organizations (ASOs) is the name given to a wide range of community-based, nongovernmental organizations which provide services to people living with AIDS. They vary widely.

In some organizations, AIDS is the only focus and all activities pertain to this issue. In other goups, AIDS is one of many issues dealt with by the agency, such as the case with health centers and multiservice social service organizations. Some have large staffs, while others have small, one or two staff person, operations. Volunteers are extensively utilized by some organizations to provide direct services to patients. Others provide services with paid staff only (Cox, 1996).

ASOs emerged in the gay community and were among the first groups in society to respond effectively and positively to AIDS. Often ASOs developed because groups of friends and family members banded together to take care of loved ones. In the process of caring for one individual, it was discovered that many others would also need services. ASOs gave vital support to people affected by HIV. . . . Even though [they] may have been originally set up primarily for gay men, the majority now provide services for all people living with AIDS, including intravenous drug users, heterosexual men and women, hemophiliacs, children, people of color, and others (ibid.).

Since they were created to meet the needs of their community, ASOs are uniquely aware of, and have an understanding of, the needs of the individual at the basic community level (including housing, religious and ethnic/cultural sensitivities), for both those who are *affected* as well as those who are *infected* by the HIV/AIDS virus.

Hospice Collaboration with ASOs Is Important to Benefit the HIV/AIDS Population

> Due to the nature of the HIV/AIDS disease progression prior to needing hospice services, most AIDS patients have already accessed community care providers [ASOs]. These relationships are important to the patient and family [and significant others] and can provide a bridge or be a barrier to accessing hospice care . . . [cannot stress enough] the importance of collaborating and building bridges [with ASOs] to ensure a continuum of quality care to all persons living with AIDS ("Overview," p. 1).

Since HIV/AIDS is a chronic, long-term illness with a terminal stage, various services will be needed at different times by people living with HIV. Usually, these arrangements are made with (or through) AIDS Service Organizations. PLWAs may need education about the implications and trajectory of the illness, medical attention, help with housing, finances, legal issues, family matters, psychological support, and such. At times, PLWAs may need minimal assistance to be able to remain at home or in their own apartment—perhaps with cooking, shopping and cleaning, provided by family, significant others, agency volunteers, or homemakers and home health aides. Other PLWAs might need more supervision and some nursing care and help with acts of daily living, perhaps in supervised residences or congregate living quarters, and still others might need 24-hour skilled nursing home care, or even hospitalization. Or the same individual might need all or some of these services at different times during the progression of the illness.

> The disease progression of HIV is neither predictable nor certain. Instead it can be characterized as a "roller coaster ride," from the low of one serious opportunistic infection to the high of treatment and response, and then another dip due to the next

infection. It is not until wasting becomes apparent that the course of AIDS achieves the predictability of cancer. This may mean that a hospice program will care for someone who is fairly functional for a period of time. Uncertain disease progression requires hospice to develop professional relationships with traditional home health agencies [and other ASOs], to share patients back and forth depending on their current disease status and need. ...Dual licensure as a hospice and a home health agency can allow flexibility (Grothe, 1996).

A number of suggestions have been presented as to how Hospices and ASOs can successfully collaborate, to the benefit of PLWAs, their families, and significant others—as well as enhancing/enriching the services offered by these organizations, always focusing on the *needs* of PLWAs. This continuity of care is so important (Brenner, 1996).

- Both Hospices and ASOs need to make each other aware— as well as the larger community—of the kind and scope of their services, what they can and cannot do; to clear up misconceptions about Hospice—that patients are not "giving up hope" when they enter the Hospice program, and that the *palliative care* offered can take many forms.
- Jointly sponsor and host periodic educational and training seminars and conferences, PLWAs' support groups, and support networks for family members and significant others.
- "ASOs can teach hospices about issues pertaining to AIDS and hospices can teach ASOs about issues pertaining to death and dying. ASOs may deal with death issues on a regular basis but may still need help with understanding the continuum of hospice care. Hospice staff ... may benefit by learning about the psychosocial dynamics of patients with HIV. **It is important not to assume that staff from ASOs and hospices understand the working of the other organization** (Cox, 1996)."
- ASOs can update Hospices about the status of HIV/AIDS in the community; and can be a valuable resource for Hospices, conerning information and services for PLWAs, their families, and significant others.
- Cox (1996) suggests that:

1. Hospices locate the ASOs in their area, find out who their clients/patients are, and the services provided to them;
2. Work together to provide a smooth, uncomplicated transition from the ASO to the Hospice program (if and when appropriate);
3. Work out agreements between the agencies as to who will be responsible for what services; and
4. Be in close communication regarding issues of mutual concern.

- Networking and collaborating with Hospice will enable the ASOs to continue their connection with PLWAs. The patient/family, and significant others will be assured of continued support from their contacts in the ASO (a relationship that developed over the course of the HIV/AIDS disease). This works well when Hospice invites and welcomes member(s) of ASOs (who have been part of the PLWAs support over the previous length of the illness), to become part of the Hospice interdisciplinary team and give active input and feedback in helping to create and implement the Hospice patient/family plan of care. This can nurture and expand relationships that can be beneficial for *all*.
- Hospice can use "partners," and this relationship can help alleviate some of the financial burden placed both on the Hospice and the ASO.
- It is critical to work together in addressing the complex issues involved in, and the barriers to, *permanency planning for the surviving children, whether infected or affected,* and to try to complete the process before the surviving parent becomes incapacitated and dies.
- The Long Island Association for AIDS Care, Inc. (LIAAC) addresses the levels of financial benefits and entitlements available to people living with AIDS, and how these can affect their children. "The problem is, however, that most of these benefits disappear upon an infected parent's death, leaving newly constructed families with an immediate and considerable financial loss. . . . The vast gap between the financial help given to infected and affected individuals once again reappears in the stipends given to foster parents.

Foster care parents (on Long Island) who take in an *adolescent living with AIDS* receive a stipend of $1,231 per month, while those who care for an *affected adolescent*, who may require significant support and services to deal with a variety of issues, receive less than half that amount—about $500. Again, this glaring gap should be closed before too many children and young adults are allowed to fall through (Reynolds, 1995)."

The importance of ASOs [and Hospices] working together, during the "anticipatory grief" and bereavement components of their programs, is further illustrated when a grandmother took over the care of two bereaved young girls. She told LIAAC interviewers:

When [my daughter] was alive, she and the kids had case managers and social workers from a couple of different agencies, they got meals delivered to the house, special financial help and [my daughter] had the support of other HIV-positive women she met at the clinic. Now that she's gone, so is all that help. I feel like I'm all by myself, left to pick up the pieces. To be honest, I'm probably not doing a great job, because I'm having a hard time, myself (Reynolds, 1995).

References

Brenner, Paul R., Exec. Dir., Jacob Perlow Hospice (New York: Private communication, May 1996).

Cox, Harold, "AIDS Service Organizations," in *Resource Manual for Providing Hospice Care to People Living with AIDS* (Arlington, VA: National Hospice Organization [NHO Resource Committee], 1996), pp. 41-3.

Grothe, Thomas, "Clinical Issues of HIV/AIDS in Hospice," *Resource Manual*, pp. 2-8.

"Overview," *Resource Manual*, p. 1.

Reynolds, Jeffrey L., writer and editor, *Reclaiming Lost Voices: Children Orphaned by HIV/AIDS in Suburbia* (Huntington Station, NY: Long Island Association for AIDS Care [LIAAC], August, 1995), pp. 71-3.

Q: Can you suggest some informative reading material about HIV/AIDS?

There are a number of "scriptographic booklets" that provide pertinent information about HIV/AIDS in an easy-to-ready for-mat. Some titles are also published in a Spanish edition.

"AIDS: An African American Woman's Story"
"AIDS: Women Get It Too"
"Anyone Can Get AIDS"
"About Hospice Under Medicare"
"Caring for People with AIDS"
"Cristina's Story About HIV—for Hispanic/Latina Women"
"HIV and AIDS: A Gay Man's Story"
"My Brother Got AIDS—An African American Man's Story."
"My Family Never Talked About AIDS—A Hispanic/Latino Man's Story"
"Talking with Your Child About AIDS—from Pre-School Through High School"
"What Everyone Should Know About AIDS"
"What Men in the Gay Community Should Know About AIDS"
"What People Over 50 Need to Know About HIV and AIDS"
"When A Loved One Has HIV"
"Why You Should Be Informed About AIDS"
"Women, HIV and AIDS—Facts for Life"

The above booklets can be ordered either from

National Hospice Organization, Inc.
1901 North Moore Street, Suite 901
Arlington, VA 22209
Hospice Helpline: 1-(800)-658-8898

or directly from the publisher:

Channing L. Bete Co., Inc.
200 State Road
South Deerfield, MA 01373
1-(800)-628-7733

Sharon Rennert, et al., *AIDS and Persons with Developmental Disabilities: The Legal Perspective* (Washington, DC: American Bar Association, the ABA Center on Children and the Law, and the Commission on the Mentally Disabled, 1989). For a copy of the above and any further information, write to:

> American Bar Association
> 1800 M Street, N.W.
> Washington, DC 20036
> (202) 331-2256

Robert W. Buckingham, *Among Friends: Hospice Care for the Person with AIDS* (Amherst, NY: Prometheus Books, 1992). According to *Choice in Dying News* (Summer 1992), 1(2):8, "A practical guide to providing Hospice care for AIDS patients, this book also describes the history and philosophy of Hospice; it could be useful reading for patients and families as well as caregivers."

"AIDS and the Hospice Community," *The Hospice Journal* (1991), 7(1/2). Special issue, Madalon O'Rawe Amenta, et al., eds. The official journal of the National Hospice Organization, this publication, issued four times a year, presents information concerning the physical, psychosocial, and pastoral care of the dying. Copies can be ordered from the publisher.

> The Haworth Press
> 10 Alice Street
> Binghamton, NY 13904-1580
> 1-(800)342-9678

National Hospice Organization, *Resource Manual for Providing Hospice Care to People Living with AIDS* (Arlington, VA: NHO 1994-1995 AIDS Resource Committee, 1996). "This *Manual* is a compilation of perceptions, experiences, expertise and perspectives on the continuum of care for persons with AIDS." Section III lists *major resources* in five categories: National Organizations, Selected AIDS-Related Databases, Selected AIDS-Related Electronic Bulletin Boards and Internet Resources, State Resources, and Recommended Reading. Can be ordered from the NHO.

Children and AIDS

Dane, Barbara O., and Carol Levin, eds., *AIDS and the New Orphans* (Westport, CT: Auburn House, 1994).

Geballe, Shelley, et al., eds., *The Forgotten Children of the AIDS Epidemic* (New Haven, CT: Yale University Press, 1995).

Levin, Carol, and Gary L. Stein, *Orphans of the HIV Epidemic* (New York: The Orphan Project, 1994).

Reynolds, Jeffrey L., writer and editor, *Reclaiming Lost Voices: Children Orphaned by HIV/AIDS in Suburbia* (Huntington Station, NY: Long Island Association for AIDS Care, Inc. [LIAAC], August, 1995). This study was funded through a 1994-1995 grant from the NY State Legislature and administered by the State Department of Health. Can be ordered from

LIAAC
PO Box 2859
Huntington Station, NY 11746
(516) 385-2437

5
ADMINISTRATION

1. Who can be referred to a Hospice program? Who can make these referrals?

2. If the patient or family is not sure if the patient is ready for Hospice care at this time, can they call the Hospice for information?

3. What needs to be in place before the patient/family is admitted to the Hospice?

4. What do the patient and family promise to provide the Hospice program before admission?

5. What is the agreement that Hospice makes to patients and families?

6. What services will be provided to the patient or family by the Hospice?

7. Does the patient or family make direct payment to the Hospice staff for services rendered? Can Hospice staff accept gifts from the patient or family?

8. What happens to a patient who no longer meets the admission criteria but wants to remain connected to the Hospice? Can the patient re-enter the Hospice program at a later date?

9. Is the Hospice staff supervised?

Q: Who can be referred to a Hospice program? Who can make these referrals?

Any patient with a terminal illness, child or adult, is a candidate for Hospice care. The majority of Hospice patients have cancer, but patients with end-stage chronic diseases such as congestive heart disease, chronic obstructive pulmonary disease, cystic fibrosis, Alzheimer's Disease, renal failure, and AIDS also can be served in a Hospice program, all benefiting from compassionate palliative and supportive care.

Patients can refer themselves to a Hospice program. Referrals can be made by families, friends, clergy, health care professionals—physicians, nurses, social workers, hospital discharge planners—and other health care providers and interested agencies.

Q: If the patient or family is not sure the patient is ready for Hospice care, can they call the Hospice for information?

Yes, the Hospice staff will share its expertise with the patient and family. This may include assistance in exploring options of care, support in recognition and awareness of diagnosis and prognosis, facilitation of communication, counseling for patient or family members prior to need for full Hospice services, and bereavement counseling for families that have not had Hospice care.

By providing guidance prior to admission eligibility, the Hospice staff can help the patient and family make informed decisions when the time does come for admission into the Hospice program.

Q: What needs to be in place before the patient/family is admitted to the Hospice?

In order for the patient to be admitted to the Hospice program, the following must be in place: (1) the patient meets the general admission criteria; (2) the patient and/or designated primary caregiver and the patient's attending physician acknowledge that the need or desire for treatment and services *not* defined as palliative would mean a formal loss of Hospice benefits; (3) the patient and attending physician agree that the Hospice plan of care will be followed, regardless of where the patient is located—whether at home, in the hospital, or in a nursing home.

Referrals will be handled by the assigned admissions staff person, possibly a nurse or social worker, who will conduct pre-admission data-gathering meetings and conversations with referred patients, family members, significant others, primary care persons, and attending physicians. Admission decisions will be handled by the assigned admissions person, with the approval of the patient care coordinator, the medical director, and social worker. The medical director must concur with the primary physician's prognosis of a life expectancy of approximately six months or less. The criteria for admission set forth by Hospice will be used for admission decisions. Once a decision is made to admit a patient/family to the

Hospice program, the fully informed consent of the primary physician, the patient, and one responsible family member shall be obtained (if there is family present and willing to participate). See Appendix A, Figure 4 (Letter from Hospice to New Patient's Attending Physician); Figure 5 (Attending Physician Authorization).

Q:What do the patient and family promise to provide the Hospice program before admission?

The patient and family must provide specific information and agree to certain conditions prior to admission to Hospice. This is essential to enable Hospice staff to address the needs and provide appropriate care for the patient, family, and significant others during the course of the illness. See Appendix A, Figure 6 (Patient/Family Consent Form).

Q: What is the agreement that Hospice makes to patients and families?

Hospice agrees to the following:

- To accept and incorporate orders of the attending physician in the Hospice plan of care.*
- To follow the wishes and desires of the patient in developing the Hospice plan of care.*
- To coordinate and maintain in writing an individual patient plan of care, incorporating the medical, social, emotional, and spiritual needs expressed by the patient, family, and attending physician.*
- To provide in-home nursing care when needed by the patient, or as indicated in the plan of care.*
- To provide counseling, support and relief to family members as needed, or indicated in the plan of care.*
- To provide direct spiritual counseling or assistance in obtaining such spiritual counseling as needed or indicated in the plan of care.*
- To provide specific treatment as needed for palliation (may include speech, physical therapy, occupational therapy, audiology, dietary counsel) or as indicated in the plan of care.*

- To provide volunteer services for the comfort, company, homemaking tasks, or pleasure of the patient and/or family as needed or indicated in the plan of care.*
- To provide equipment and supplies necessary for the patient's comfort and care as indicated by the plan of care.*
- To provide drugs and biologicals necessary for palliative treatment of the patient's terminal illness as indicated by the plan of care.* (See also "What is meant by 'drugs and biologicals' used in a Medicare certified Hospice program?" in Chapter 9.)
- To determine appropriate location for treatment in the event the patient's condition and plan of care requires inpatient care.*

Q: What services will be provided to the patient or family by the Hospice?

Hospice services include:

- Nursing care provided by or under the supervision of a registered nurse.
- Nursing care made available on a twenty-four (24) hour basis.
- Medical social services provided by a social worker under the direction of a physician.
- Physician services performed by a doctor of medicine or osteopathy serving as the Hospice medical director, and physician member of the interdisciplinary team.
- Counseling services provided to the terminally ill individual and the family members, or other persons caring for the patient (including dietary counseling) for the purpose of:

  a. Training the individual's family or other caregiver to provide care, and/or
  b. Helping the individual and those caring for him/her to adjust to the individual's approaching death.

---

* All items so marked are required for those patients electing to use Medicare Hospice Benefits.

- Short-term inpatient care in a hospital or skilled nursing facility, as indicated in the patient's Hospice plan of care for pain control or acute or chronic symptom management.
- Inpatient respite care to provide temporary relief for the patient's family or other person(s) caring for the patient at home.
- Respite care will be provided on an occasional basis and only for brief periods of time—usually five days or less.
- Medical appliances and supplies, including drugs and biologicals:

    a. Drugs needed primarily for the relief of pain and symptom control related to the individual's terminal illness will be provided when indicated in the patient's Hospice plan of care and with appropriate physician orders;

    b. Appliances, including durable medical equipment (such as wheelchairs, commodes, hospital beds), as well as other self-help and personal comfort items related to the palliation of management of the patient's terminal illness, as indicated in the patient's Hospice plan of care, will be provided by Hospice for use in the patient's home while he/she is under Hospice care.

- Home health aide services and homemaker services will be provided as indicated in patient's Hospice plan of care, including:

    a. Household services to maintain a safe and sanitary environment in areas of the home used by the patient and essential to the comfort and cleanliness of the patient;

    b. Assistance in personal care and services to enable the individual to carry out the Hospice plan of care.

    (These aide services will be provided under the general supervision of a registered nurse.)

- Physical therapy, occupational therapy, audiology, and speech-language pathology services will be provided for purposes of symptom control or to enable patient to maintain activities of daily living (ADL) and basic functional skills.

- Nursing care will be provided on a continuous basis for as much as twenty-four (24) hours/day during periods of crisis* as necessary to achieve palliation or management of acute medical symptoms, while maintaining the patient at home. (This continuous care will be predominantly nursing care with either homemakers or home health aides supplementing the nursing care.)
- Bereavement counseling will be provided to the patient's family after his/her death, up to at least one year following the death of the patient. "Anticipatory Grief Counseling" may be provided prior to the death of the patient. (See "What Is Meant by 'Anticipatory Grief'?" in Chapter 11.)

Q: Does the patient or family make direct payment to the Hospice staff for services rendered?

Hospice employees and volunteers are prohibited from receiving payment from any patient, family, or party other than Hospice for services provided as part of the Hospice program or from splitting or sharing fees between a referral agency/facility or individual and the Hospice.

Occasionally, individuals or groups express appreciation for services provided with an offer of a gift to a member of the Hospice staff or a volunteer. They may *not* accept a gift in excess of $10 in value. It is appropriate to point out that a gift or donation to Hospice would be acceptable: perhaps a memorial gift or one in honor of a special occasion, or to help support a program of Hospice that was of great help to the patient or family.

Q: What happens to a patient who no longer meets the admission criteria but wants to remain connected to the

---

* Note: Nursing care, physician services, drugs, and biologicals are routinely available on a 24-hour basis. All other services are available on a 24-hour basis to the extent necessary to meet the needs of individuals as indicated on the patient's Hospice plan of care.

Hospice? Can a patient re-enter the Hospice program at a later date?

When a medical assessment indicates that the patient's disease is temporarily stabilized, symptoms are controlled, and the patient is stable psychosocially, the patient and family may agree to be declared "inactive" after meeting with the physician and Hospice staff.

When the Hospice team sees there is potential for inactive status, the physician assesses the patient's condition and determines that the patient's disease is temporarily stable. Then both the physician and appropriate Hospice team members meet with the patient and family to explain the change in status and exactly what it means to them.

Another agency may be suggested for interim services at this time. Since a patient may re-enter the Hospice program when it is appropriate, it is important for a member of the Hospice team to maintain regular contact with the patient and family until they return to active status in the Hospice program.

Q: Is the Hospice staff supervised?

Each staff member of the Hospice program has an identified supervisor who is responsible for the clarification of any information related to Hospice policies and procedures. The supervisor makes assignments and is accessible to the staff. The supervisor of the Hospice is skilled in basic human relations and personnel management, and is sensitive to the emotional investment and stress experienced by staff as they care for their terminally ill patients, family, and significant others.

6
ADVANCE DIRECTIVES

1. How can the patient and family be assured their wishes will be made known to the Hospice team ("Advance Directives")?

2. What is a "Do-Not-Resuscitate Order"?

3. Does the Hospice program require a do-not-resuscitate order prior to admission?

4. What is a "Health Care Proxy"?

5. What is a "Living Will?" How can it affect the care of the Hospice patient?

6. What is a "Durable Power of Attorney"?

7. What do these "Advance Directives" look like?

Q: How can the patient and family be assured their wishes will be made known to the Hospice team ("Advance Directives")?

Some advance directives have been mandated by both federal and state laws, including the "Patient Self-Determination Act." Hospice programs,

... pursuant to applicable federal and state laws, are committed to supporting an adult patient's right to make decisions concerning his or her health care and to honoring these advance directives relating to the provision of such care when the patient is incapacitated and unable to direct his or her own health care.

Advance directives are written instructions relating to the provision of health care such as a health care proxy, a consent to the issuance of an order not to resuscitate, or a living will. Patients may also give specific instructions orally by discussing, in a clear and convincing manner, their treatment wishes with physicians, family members or others.

It is the Hospice's policy to ensure that all patients and families are informed of their rights and to support its patients as they exercise their rights to formulate advance directives ("Advance Directives," 1991).

Discussions about a living will, durable power of attorney, the health care proxy, and do-not-resuscitate orders ensure that the patient's family and significant others, as well as the Hospice staff, will respect the patient's requests and incorporate them into the development and updating of the plan of care.

Since these discussions may evoke many emotions, it is essential that they be handled in a sensitive manner and be given time to come to a conclusion.

Hospice staff are well aware that frequently a number of discussions about these advance directives may be necessary over a period of time to give patients and families the opportunity to truly understand, absorb, and integrate this knowledge. Thus, they are given the opportunity to come to an informed conclusion with which they will be comfortable.

Some people may feel it is morbid to discuss these issues, yet many patients and families have said that once advance directives were in place, they had more time for personal issues and there was less confusion and conflict when decisions had to be made during the dying process.

The National Hospice Organization "Hospice Fact Sheet" (1995) states:

> . . . Ninety-eight percent of hospices require signed "informed consent" for all patients; only 40 percent require DNR [do not resuscitate] orders for all patients. In some states, the Patient Self-Determination Act makes it a violation of federal law to require a DNR order as part of the admission criteria.

References

Advance Directives (New York: St. Luke's/Roosevelt Hospital Center, 1991).

Hospice Fact Sheet (Arlington, VA: National Hospice Organization, updated October 10, 1995).

Q: What is a "Do-Not-Resuscitate Order"?

(*The following questions and answers are quoted from the New York State Department of Health.*)

A do-not-resuscitate (DNR) order in the patient's medical chart instructs the medical staff not to try to revive the patient if breathing or heartbeat has stopped. This means physicians, nurses, and others will not initiate such emergency procedures as mouth-to-mouth resuscitation, external chest compression, electric shock, insertion of a tube to open the patient's airway, injection of medication into the heart, or open-chest heart massage.

If the patient is in a nursing home, a DNR order instructs the staff not to perform emergency resuscitation and not to transfer the patient to a hospital for such procedures.

What are the advantages and disadvantages of CPR?

Cardiopulmonary resuscitation (CPR), when successful, restores heartbeat and breathing and enables a patient to resume his or her previous lifestyle. In other cases, CPR may fail to restore basic life functions or only partially succeed, leaving the patient brain damaged or otherwise impaired.

The success of CPR depends on the patient's overall medical condition and level of functioning before hospitalization. Age alone is not a predictor of success, although illnesses and frailties associated with advanced age often result in less successful outcomes.

Are DNR orders ethically acceptable?

It is widely recognized by health care professionals, clergy, lawyers, and others that DNR orders are medically and ethically appropriate under certain circumstances. For some patients, CPR offers more burdens than benefits and may be contrary to the patient's wishes.

How can I make my wishes about DNR known?

An adult patient in a hospital or nursing home [or Hospice] can consent to a DNR order orally, as long as two witnesses are present. One witness must be a physician. You can also make your wishes known before or during hospitalization in writing, before any two adults who must sign your statement as witnesses. A living will may be used to convey these wishes, as long as it is properly witnessed.

You can specify that you want a DNR order only under certain circumstances (such as if you become terminally ill or permanently unconscious) or that you wish only specific CPR procedures performed, such as mouth-to-mouth breathing but not open-heart massage.

Before making a decision about CPR, you should speak with your physician about your overall health and the benefits and burdens CPR would provide for you. A full and early discussion between you and your doctor can avoid later misunderstandings.

If I request a DNR order, is my physician bound to honor my wishes?

If you don't want to be resuscitated and you request a DNR order, your physician must either:

- enter the order in your chart; or
- transfer responsibility for your care to another physician; or
- refer the matter to a dispute mediation system in the hospital or nursing home. The mediation system is only authorized to mediate disputes; it cannot overrule your decision.

If mediation has not resolved the dispute within 72 hours, your physician must enter the order or transfer you to the care of another physician.

What happens if I do not have the capacity to decide for myself?

You are presumed by law to be mentally capable of deciding about CPR unless two physicians, or a court, determines that you no longer have the capacity to make the decision. You will be informed of this determination if you are able to understand it, and no DNR order will be written if you object.

If I do not have the mental capacity to make a decision about CPR and do not leave instructions in advance, who will decide?

If you lose the capacity to decide and did not leave advance instructions, a DNR order can be entered only with the consent of someone chosen by you in advance, or by a family member or another person with a close personal relationship to you. The person highest on the following list will decide on your behalf:

- a person you have selected to decide about resuscitation;
- a court appointed guardian (if there is one);
- your closest relative;
- a close friend.

How can I select someone to decide for me?

If you are a patient in a hospital or nursing home, you can appoint a person orally, with two witnesses present.

You can also appoint someone during or in advance of hospitalization by stating your wishes in writing and signing that statement with any two adults present. The adults must also sign your written statement.

Under what circumstances can a family member or close friend consent to a DNR order?

A family member or close friend can consent to a DNR order only when you are unable to decide for yourself and:

- you have a terminal condition; or
- you are permanently unconscious; or
- CPR would be medically futile; or
- CPR would impose an extraordinary burden on you, given your medical condition and the expected outcome of resuscitation.

Anyone deciding for you must base the decision on your wishes, including your religious and moral beliefs, or if your wishes are not known, on your best interest.

What if members of my family disagree?

They can ask for the matter to be mediated. Your physician will request mediation if he or she is aware of any disagreement among family members.

What if I lose the capacity to decide and do not have anyone who can decide on my behalf?

A DNR order can be entered only if two physicians conclude that CPR would be medically useless or if a court approves the DNR order. It would be best if you discussed the matter with your physician and left instructions in advance.

Who can consent to a DNR order for children?

A DNR order can be entered in the record for a patient under the age of eighteen only with the consent of the patient's parent or guardian. If the minor has the capacity to decide, the minor's consent is also required for a DNR order.

What happens to a DNR order if I am transferred from a nursing home to a hospital or vice versa?

The health facility where you are sent can continue the DNR order but is not obligated to do so. If the order is not continued, you or anyone who decided on your behalf will be informed and can request that the order be entered again.

What happens if I change my mind after I consent to a DNR order?

You or anyone who consents to a DNR order on your behalf can withdraw that consent at any time by informing your physician, nurses, or others of the decision (*Do Not Resuscitate Orders,* 1989).

Reference

Do Not Resuscitate Orders (A Guide for Patients and Families) (Albany, NY: New York State Department of Health, February 1989).

Q: Does the Hospice program require a do-not-resuscitate order prior to admission?

Hospice programs may differ in their admission criteria and may or may not require a signed do-not-resuscitate (DNR) order prior to or at the time of admission into the Hospice program.

The DNR order is a directive that needs to be discussed carefully when the patient and family are reviewing their options for Hospice care. By working together with the Hospice team, the patient, family, and significant others will gain insights and have a clearer picture of their options as well as a better understanding of the focus of the patient's individual plan of care. They then may decide that the DNR order is appropriate for them.

When signed, authorization for Hospice DNR records is placed in the patient's medical record file. Three examples of these are shown in Appendix A, Figures 7, 8, and 9. (*Hospice Operations Manual*, 1990.)

Reference

Hospice Operations Manual (Hempstead, NY: Long Island Foundation for Hospice Care and Research, Inc., 1990), pp. 432-4.

Q: What is a "Health Care Proxy"?

In order to insure that each patient's wishes are known, understood, and honored, as part of the Patient Self-Determination Act, a patient has a right to execute a "Health Care Proxy" (*Health Care Proxy*, 1991). This means that you give the person you choose as your agent the authority to make all health care decisions for you, except to the extent you say otherwise. *Health care* means any treatment, service, or procedure to diagnose or treat your physical or mental condition.

Unless the patient states otherwise, this person will be allowed to make all health care decisions for the patient, including decisions to remove or provide life-sustaining treatment. It is important that this proxy knows your wishes about artificial nutrition and hydration. Your health care proxy will start to make decisions for you when the doctors decide you are unable to make health care decisions for yourself.

This is another means whereby the Hospice program will know the wishes of the patient and be able to assist the individual designated as the health care proxy in honoring these directives. Thus, the patient continues to be involved in the decision-making process, even though no longer competent.

Reference

Health Care Proxy: Guidelines (Albany, NY: New York State Department of Health, 1991).

Q: What is a "Living Will"? How can it affect the care of the Hospice patient?

A living will is a person's statement that he or she wishes to be allowed to die naturally and not be kept alive by artificial means or heroic measures. Signed by the patient when mentally competent, the living will authorizes designated others to decide for the patient if he or she is unable to make decisions.

Living wills authorize medications for the relief of pain and suffering, with the knowledge that supportive comfort care will be provided. This document may include suggestions for the person designated to make binding decisions. It also may mention specific types of treatment that would be objected to, such as mechanical respiration, cardiopulmonary resuscitation, and nasogastric tube feedings. The living will also may have options for other situations, such as organ donations and death at home rather than in the hospital.

A living will may be revoked at any time, as long as the patient is mentally competent at the time of revocation. The patient is free to disagree at any time with the terms of the living will and make revisions at will.

The living will is another advance directive to assist the patient, the families, and significant others in the knowledge that the wishes of the patient will be known to the Hospice staff and that these wishes will be incorporated into the patient's plan of care.

Each state in the United States has its own legal requirements, and a living will may not be legally recognized in all states. However, it makes health care institutions and courts aware of the wishes of the patient. This is invaluable if some legal matter needs to be addressed in decision making at a future date.

Reference

Annas, G., et al. *The Rights of Doctors, Nurses and Allied Health Professionals* (New York: Avon Books, 1981).

Q: What is a "Durable Power of Attorney"?

One means of safeguarding the incompetent patient's wishes through an advance directive is the durable power of attorney. Ordinary power of attorney is in effect only as long as the person remains competent and able to make informed decisions. With the onset of mental incompetency, ordinary power of attorney lapses.

Durable power of attorney, however, is *not* automatically voided when the patient becomes incapacitated. This document may be worded in such a way that it will not take effect until and unless the patient becomes incompetent, at which time the designated person (or persons) makes health care treatment decisions *and* assumes responsibility.

Also called a "medical power of attorney," most become operative when your physician concludes that you are unable to make your own medical decisions. If you regain the ability to make decisions, your agent cannot continue to act for you. Many states have additional requirements that apply only to decisions about life support. For example, before your agent can refuse a life-sustaining treatment on your behalf, a second physician may have to confirm your doctor's assessment that you are incapable of making treatment decisions.

Patients/families, before or after admission to the Hospice program, may explore the options of durable power of attorney in order to encourage the patients to have their wishes respected, should they become incompetent to make these decisions (*Ethics Committee*, 1985).

Reference

Ethics Committee: Decisions in Hospice (Arlington, VA: National Hospice Organization, 1985).

Q: What do these "Advance Directives" look like?

Since each state has different legal requirements, it is important that your documents be legally sound and conform to the laws in your particular state.

For example, according to a New York elder law attorney Arlene Kane, RN, "Although New York does not have a specific statute recognizing living wills, as many other states do, New York courts have upheld the right of self-determination through its common law."

Advance directive documents specific for your state can be requested free of charge from local hospitals, state bar associations, and state health departments, as well as from Choice in Dying, 200 Varick Street, New York, NY 10014. Tel.: (212) 366-5540; FAX (212) 366-5337; or 1-800-989-WILL.

7
AMERICAN ACADEMY OF HOSPICE AND PALLIATIVE MEDICINE

1. What can the patient and family expect from their attending physician who understands the Hospice philosophy?

2. Does Hospice care include euthanasia or assisted suicide?

3. Are there physicians in the United States today who are active advocates for Hospice/Palliative Care as part of mainstream medicine?

Q: What can the patient and family expect from their attending physician, who understands the Hospice philosophy?

The patient and family can expect the following from the physician, according to Dr. Robert Miller.

Physicians have an obligation to promote the life and health of the patient and to relieve suffering. If these goals are in conflict, the preference of the patient takes priority. For a patient with an incurable disease, quality of life may be chosen as the most important goal. The physician must treat for pain and symptom control with the same degree of intensity and urgency as accorded any other medical condition....

Patient autonomy is not an end in itself. Most patients prefer to have their physicians advise and assist them in making important health care decisions. An important goal is encouraging a doctor-patient relationship based on honesty and true caring so that patients feel confident that their best interests will always be foremost....

The physician has an obligation to provide, within the best of his ability, as much medical care as is available, and appropriate to benefit the patient according to the wishes of the patient.

Reference

Miller, Dr. Robert, First President of the American Academy of Hospice and Palliative Medicine (formerly the Academy of Hospice Physicians), Medical Director of St. Anthony's Cancer Care Center, Board Member of The Hospice of the Florida Suncoast [formerly Hospice Care, Inc.], Largo, FL.

Q: Does Hospice care include euthanasia or assisted suicide?

Hospice care is comfort care incorporating palliative medicine, pain control, and symptom management. This care does not prolong the dying process, nor does it shorten life. However, survival often is prolonged through the patient becoming more comfortable. Comfort often enhances function and, by improving function of the patient, Hospices often provide quality time for dying patients and their families.

Hospice care does not include euthanasia or assisted suicide.

Physicians have an obligation to consider the possible harm which might result from treatment. Professional recommendations regarding the likely benefit and potential harm of various treatment options should be offered for the patient's consideration. Therapy designed and intended to relieve suffering in a terminally ill patient is ethically acceptable even if it secondarily shortens survival. Interventions that have the primary goal of shortening human life such as physician-assisted suicide and active euthanasia run counter to the accepted role of the physician and have not been considered ethical within the doctor-patient relationship.

Active efforts to shorten survival also run counter to the goal of the hospice movement which recognizes that if adequate symptom control is attained, the final period before death may be very significant and meaningful to both patient and family. It is also recognized that the goals of developing and improving optimal palliative care may be compromised in a society that promotes or legalizes assisted suicide or euthanasia.

The American Academy of Hospice and Palliative Medicine makes a clear "Position Statement" on this ethical issue:

We stand in fellowship with all those who are striving to diminish the pain and suffering of the dying.

As hospice physicians involved in the compassionate care of the terminally ill, we have observed that competent palliative care usually relieves the pain and suffering of terminally ill persons and their families.

In the current debate we oppose legalization of euthanasia (mercy killing) and assisted suicide. We call instead for public policy changes that ensure genuine access to comprehensive hospice services for all dying patients—regardless of socioeconomic status, age or diagnosis. (Position Statement, 1991)

In the article "The Right to Die Rightly," by Rev. Bill Wallace, the National Hospice Organization's position is quoted.

Euthanasia is different in kind, not degree from treatments that allow death to occur or even those which unintentionally hasten it. No patient need die in pain. Although the ideal goal of palliative care is to maximize comfort and function, effective symptom control in some patients causes forfeiture of cognitive function, discontinuation of eating and drinking, suppression of cough reflex, and depression of respiration. These unintended consequences may hasten death caused by the underlying disease; they do not of themselves directly cause death.

As Rev. Wallace states:

Hospice continues to pioneer the development of state-of-the-art pain control...developing better ways for dying persons to describe and locate their pain for caregivers...teach caregivers to assess and treat the spiritual, social and emotional elements of pain, as well as its physical causes. Physicians write range doses and medicate "this side" of the pain threshold so dying persons can avoid being controlled or influenced by pain.

We must push harder to give back what medicine surrendered in its ascent up the mountain of high tech—the caring relationship which must form the basis of encounters between clinicians and patients.

References

Academy of Hospice Physicians, "A Position Statement," St. Petersburg, FL, 1991.

Miller, R. J., "Basic Ethical Principles and Terminal Care," *Newsletter: Physician Bulletin* (Largo, FL.: The Hospice of the Florida Suncoast), (Summer 1991), 4(2):2.

Wallace, Rev. B., "The Right to Die Rightly," *Hospice Magazine* (Arlington, VA: National Hospice Organization), (Summer 1992), pp. 11, 28.

Q: Are there physicians in the United States today who are active advocates for Hospice/Palliative Care as part of mainstream medicine?

Yes. Many physicians are working with the American Academy of Hospice and Palliative Medicine to carry out their mission, which has five major components:

- Take an active role in the future education of physicians, informing and educating practicing physicians about appropriate care of the dying patient, bringing the hospice philosophy of care into the medical school curriculum, and participating in research aimed at improving all aspects of patient care;
- Play the role of ombudsman in protecting the rights and personal autonomy of dying patients and their families, and see that their needs are not neglected or curtailed;
- Provide a format that supports and promotes physicians with an interest in palliative care medicine;
- Have a strong voice in the future dialogue concerning local and national policy that will impact on palliative care, and collaborate with other members of the hospice team in promoting palliative care;

- Take an active part in the philosophic and ethical discussions concerning the role of the physician, as the role is constantly being redefined in an ever changing society.

According to Dale Smith, Executive Director, the American Academy of Hospice and Palliative Medicine would like to see "palliative medicine" accepted as a medical specialty.

Palliative medicine is about caring for people. It acknowledges that dying does not denote a failure to provide quality medical care, but rather an acceptance that the goal of a course of treatment must shift from curing to caring. The ultimate development of palliative medicine as a recognized medical specialty will ensure the availability of quality medical education in this field at all levels. Further, reimbursement mechanisms will be tailored to ensure that proper care of the terminally ill will not only be available to the few possessing significant personal resources, but to all who rightfully demand the quality and dignity of such services.

(See also "History of Hospice," Chapter 1.)

Reference

Academy of Hospice Physicians, "Mission Statement," St. Petersburg, FL, 1992.

Smith, Dale C., Executive Director, Academy of Hospice Physicians (Gainesville, FL: Private communication, November 1995).

8
PHYSICIANS ADDRESS ISSUES
OF PALLIATIVE CARE

1. What marks the beginning of terminal illness?

2. What does the physician have to offer the terminally ill patient and family? What is "Palliative Care"?

3. How can the physician facilitate the patient's and family's well-being through Hospice care?

4. What are the advantages and disadvantages of Hospice care for the terminally ill patient and family?

5. Will the patient have to change doctors? What is the relationship of the patient's attending physician and the Hospice physician? What is the role of the attending physician when the patient is in the Hospice program? Do Hospice physicians really make house calls? What are some of the factors that influence the attending physician to relinquish care when the patient is admitted to the Hospice program?

6. How does the patient's attending physician feel about giving a six-month prognosis for the Medicare certified Hospice program? How does the attending physician feel about referring a patient to Hospice? Why do some physicians wait until the death of the patient is imminent before referring the patient to Hospice?

7. Does Hospice force religion or spirituality on its patients?

8. What is the importance of symptom control in terminal care?

9. How can the physical pain of a terminally ill patient be adequately alleviated?

10. Will I become addicted to narcotics if I take them for pain? Will they hasten the end? Does Hospice use too much morphine?

11. How does the Hospice physician feel about honoring patient and family requests concerning "patient self-determination": the health care proxy, do-not-resuscitate orders, living wills, and the durable power of attorney?

12. What happens at the time of the patient's death in a Hospice program?

Q: What marks the beginning of terminal illness?

While some would say that we are all born to die, which makes us all terminally ill from the day we are born, we in the United States, by federal mandate, have designated the last six months of life as appropriate for Hospice care. This artificial designation has proved problematic because there is so much variation among individual patients that accurate prognostication is extremely difficult, if not impossible, on a case-by-case basis.

For some physicians, it is extremely difficult to determine when an illness becomes terminal, especially in chronic illness where there is no clearly defined demarcation between a preterminal or terminal condition. Some patients are really on a continuum without sharply defined periods of deterioration, often right up to the time of death. When it becomes clear to the physician that all available treatments for a patient's life-threatening illness are ineffective for cure, it is time to acknowledge that the patient has entered the terminal phase of illness (Schneiderman, Jecker, and Jonsen, 1991). Some physicians are very reluctant to make that medical judgment, and even more reluctant to share that information with the patients, their families, and their loved ones. There is a tendency for physicians to view inability to cure as a failure and to feel uncomfortable telling the patient that there are no further curative options available. Good medical care does not end when the physician is no longer able to cure disease.

Frequently, the patient or family recognizes the ineffectiveness of treatment but may be reluctant to speak about it with the attending physician. Open and adequate communication among patient, family, and physician is vital in any patient-physician relationship, particularly for the patient with life-threatening illness. The patient has the right and obligation to participate in decisions regarding his or her care and medical management (Patient Rights, 1992; President's Commission, 1983). It is particularly important when those decisions involve a shift from cure to palliation and/or discussion of quality of life or life-prolonging measures. It is important to talk about realities and the options that remain. Prior to Hospice admission, the physician should share information about the appropriateness and effectiveness of treatment and may suggest consultation with another specialist for a second opinion.

Part of the recognition of terminal illness includes provision of appropriate support services for the patient and family or significant others. Often it is the family, friends, and patients themselves who make the Hospice referral for assistance with home nursing care and psychosocial support. These support services can be spiritual, psychological, and emotional, and include financial and practical concerns. Patients should be encouraged to consider advance directives such as the health care proxy, durable power of attorney, living wills, and do-not-resuscitate orders. It is also appropriate to make or update their wills, provide for care of any minor children, and complete other tasks related to end-of-life decision making.

References

Patient Rights, *Accreditation Manual for Hospitals* (1992), RI.1 and RI.1.1, pp. 1-15.

President's Commission for the Study of Ethical Problems in Medicine and Biomedical and Behavioral Research. *Deciding to forgo life-sustaining treatment: a report on the ethical, medical and legal issues in treatment decisions* (Washington, DC: Government Printing Office, 1983).

Schneiderman, L. J., N. S. Jecker, and A. R. Jonsen, "Medical Futility: Its Meaning and Ethical Implications," *Annals of Internal Medicine* (1991), 112:949-54.

Q: What does the physician have to offer the terminally ill patient and family? What is "Palliative Care"?

The terminally ill patient and family have the right to expect continued care and support from the physician and health care team. The physician will continue to evaluate the patient for ongoing and new problems, monitor symptoms, evaluate changes in the patient's condition, prescribe medication, make appropriate referrals, and communicate with the patient about his or her condition. The physician should explore the patient's wishes regarding issues such as resuscitation and control of pain, provide access to a social worker to assist with financial issues, and provide information regarding palliative care and Hospice (Brown, 1992).

The Hospice physician offers the patient and family competent palliative care, including relief from pain. This includes home care primarily, but with the potential for service in hospitals and nursing homes when appropriate.

Palliative care means "affording relief, but not cure." Robert Twycross, borrowing a quotation from Sir William Osler, defines palliative medicine as

- To cure sometimes
- To relieve often
- To comfort always.

Palliative medicine, as opposed to traditionally curative medicine, involves an ethos of caring instead of an ethos of curing. The goal is to maintain human dignity by communicating freely with patients and allowing them to participate fully in decisions regarding their care. Palliative care is goal oriented. Symptom control is provided by having a clearly defined, *patient-directed* plan of care. Hope is not taken away from the patient. Robert Twycross initiates patient contact by asking, "What do you hope will come out of this consultation?" There is no false hope of cure, but there is plenty of hope for symptom control, relief from suffering, and quality time.

References

Brown,W. W., ed., "Caring for the Terminally Ill Patient, Overview," in *Death and Dying: Working with the Life-Threatened Patient and Family* (St. Louis, MO: St. Louis University School of Medicine, 1992), pp. 83-126.

Twycross, Robert, "Why Palliative Medicine?" Estes Park, CO: Keynote Presentation, Sixth International Hospice Institute Symposium, July 20, 1990.

Q: How can the physician facilitate the patient's and family's well-being through Hospice care?

It is appropriate that the patient's attending physician share with the patient an honest assessment of his or her current condition. Together they may wish to review the past benefits of treatment and any negative side-effects. They then can discuss the alternatives of continuing an ineffective disease-oriented treatment or of shifting to a supportive, person-oriented, comfort-directed approach. The attending physician ought to be willing to share with the patient as many of the practical implications of this decision as the patient wishes to know. Included in this discussion can be an explicit statement of the physician's ongoing commitment to the patient and to the goal of maintaining his or her comfort and function at as high a level as possible. When it is clear that the patient understands the alternatives, the physician ought to give the patient time to make a decision and be available to discuss alternatives again. The attending physician also should ask about the patient's willingness to share this information with the family and take into consideration the extent to which the patient wishes the family to be involved in the decision making (Brown, 1992; Schoene-Seifert and Childress, 1986; Johnson, 1992).

When the patent has made a decision to relinquish disease-curing attempts, the physician ought to inquire about the patient's attitudes regarding quality of life. What physical, emotional, and social conditions are crucial to the patient's desire to live longer? What circumstances would the patient find so personally compromising as to be intolerable? Are there any events or goals (for example, a birth, wedding, graduation) to which the patient looks forward? (Holland, 1992).

Once the focus of treatment has shifted from cure to comfort care, it is important for the physician to talk with the patient about the possible settings in which this care might be given. Then the two of them can discuss with the patient's family the alternatives of hospital care, outpatient treatment, Hospice care, or home care. The family's desires and ability to participate in the patient's care at home or in a long-term care facility should be evaluated. The patient and family also ought to be informed about the extent to which the physician could continue to be involved in the patient's care in any of these settings.

The interdisciplinary team is the primary strength of any Hospice program. By referring a patient and family for Hospice care, the physician facilitates care for the patient physically, emotionally, mentally, and spiritually through using various team members. However, there is a role for the physician to play in the areas not traditionally recognized as the domain of the physician.

Derek Doyle discusses the role of the physician in meeting spiritual needs.

First, we can listen and then ask if that is sufficient for the patient. Often it is, but it may be the first time they have ever articulated the problem or had anyone care enough to listen....They are the ones who frighten us because we intuitively feel we should make the mistake of thinking the patient wants radical spiritual surgery or even worse, a miracle. What they want is first to hear that others have felt the same and come through it; second, that we as all-knowing doctors also have and have had our doubts; third, that we are not surprised or shocked at their revelation and view this problem in the same way as any physical or psychosocial one. They want to be assured that they are normal; that they are experiencing something common to man, familiar to us all, and in the uniqueness of their dying are not unique in their suffering (Doyle, 1992).

The physician can best facilitate Hospice care through cooperation with the interdisciplinary team, while continuing to provide the traditional physician role of medical direction and leadership. In addition to this, by providing services outside the traditional role of the physician, always continuing to compassionately care about the patient, the physician truly can facilitate a comfortable death for the patient.

References

Brown, W. W., ed., "Caring for the Adult and Family Facing Life-Threatening Illness" and "Caring for the Terminally Ill Patient," in *Death and Dying: Working with the Life-Threatened Patient and Family* (St. Louis, MO: St. Louis University School of Medicine, 1992), pp. 21-44; 83-126.

Doyle, D., "Have We Looked Beyond the Physical and Psychosocial?" *Journal of Pain and Symptom Management* (July 1992), 7(5):302-11.

Holland, J. C., "Stress and Coping: Families and Terminal Illness," in *Death and Dying: Working with the Life-Threatened Patient and Family,* W. W. Brown (ed.) (St. Louis, MO: St. Louis University School of Medicine, 1992), pp. 64-7.

Johnson, S. H., "Legal Aspects of Health Care Decision-Making," in *Death and Dying: Working with the Life-Threatened Patient and*

Family, W. W. Brown (ed.) (St. Louis, MO: St. Louis University School of Medicine, 1992), pp. 186-93.

Schoene-Seifert, B., and J. F. Childress, "How much should the cancer patient know and decide?" *CA—A Cancer Journal for Clinicians* (March-April 1986), 36(2).

Q: What are the advantages and disadvantages of Hospice care for the terminally ill patient and family?

One of the first differences among Hospices is whether or not they are full-service. Those that are certified by Medicare and Medicaid provide the entire range of services. Hospices that are not certified may not be able to offer the entire range of services. It is important for the physician making the Hospice referral to know which type of agency is involved.

The Hospice Medicare Benefit provides funding to Hospices on a *per diem* arrangement. In other words, Medicare pays the Hospice a fixed rate for each day a patient is in the Hospice program, regardless of the kind and frequency of services provided. When the patient elects the Medicare Hospice Benefit, the Hospice in turn becomes responsible for the cost of the patient's care related to the terminal illness. The Hospice Medicare Benefit includes a 5 percent patient copayment toward the cost of medication. The certified Hospice program provides supplies, durable medical equipment such as hospital beds in the home, nursing care, and hospitalizations as necessary.

Patients and families entering Hospice must be aware that the goal of Hospice is palliation and symptom relief rather than cure. Patients or family members who have not recognized that the illness is terminal and further treatment futile will be very frustrated by and unhappy in the Hospice environment. All care is symptom based, and no testing or treatment is ordered without a clear goal of symptom relief identified in the patient's plan of care.

Some patients and family members may feel uncomfortable with Hospice or view symptom-oriented care as somehow second class or incomplete. If the patient wishes to persist in disease-oriented treatment in hope of a cure or "to live as much life as possible," the physician may decide to comply with the patient's request. However, the doctor who feels morally or ethically compromised by such a course of action may discuss this with the patient, withdraw from the patient's care, and assist the patient in finding a competent physician who would be willing to continue aggressive treatment. It is far preferable, however, for the physician, patient, and family to come to agreement. The last phase of terminal illness is a poor time to change physicians and support systems.

Hospice provides excellent palliative care, most often in the patient's or family's home. Providing comfort through medical techniques of pain management and symptom relief often involves less technology than that provided in a hospital environment, usually adds to the patient's feeling of peace, and allows the patient to remain in control.

While Hospice caregivers are experts in pain and symptom control, the patient remains in control of the care he or she receives for as long as is possible. Decisions about all treatment, including potentially life-prolonging measures, are left to the patient.

The Hospice interdisciplinary team is crucial to this form of care. (See also "What Is the Interdisciplinary Team?" in Chapter 9.) In order to meet all needs of the dying and their families, multiple specialists are needed. While physicians and nurses concentrate on the medical needs of the patient, they also provide psychosocial and often spiritual support. Hospice volunteers form close personal relationships that will help sustain the patient, the family, and significant others throughout the dying and, later, the grieving process. (See also "What Do Hospice Volunteers Do?" in Chapter 10.)

Hospice care does not end with the death of the patient. In every case, bereavement follow-up and counseling is provided for a period of at least twelve months for the family. In Hospice, the patient and family are the unit of care, and for this reason the task is not complete until the family has been helped in the grieving process. (See also "How Does the Hospice Offer Bereavement Services?" in Chapter 11.)

There are no disadvantages to Hospice care other than the initial receiving and acceptance of a terminal prognosis. Unfortunately, reluctance on the part of the referring physician to communicate a terminal prognosis results in less than a third of patients who qualify for Hospice actually receiving Hospice care, according to W. W. Brown, M.D.

Emotional, physical, and spiritual comfort is the goal of Hospice care. A comfortable death is all that any human being can hope for, and that is what Hospice strives to provide (Brown, 1992).

Reference

Brown, W. W., ed., "Caring for the Terminally Ill Patient," in *Death and Dying: Working with the Life-Threatened Patient and Family* (St. Louis, MO: St. Louis University School of Medicine, 1992), pp. 85-95.

Q: Will the patient have to change doctors? What is the relationship of the patient's attending physician and the Hospice physician? What is the role of the attending physician when the patient is in the Hospice program? Do Hospice physicians really make house calls? What are some of the factors that influence the attending physician to relinquish care when the patient is admitted to the Hospice program?

These five questions have been asked frequently. Responding to them as a group gives a clearer picture of the role of both the patient's attending physician and the Hospice physician.

The Hospice Medicare Benefit provides for reimbursement to Hospices regardless of environment: the patient's home, a hospital, a nursing home, or alternative residential setting with Hospice support. The most appropriate environment for the patient is therefore always available without jeopardizing the Hospice or patient from a financial standpoint. This flexibility allows patients to move appropriately between environments without concern about losing continuity of care. The Hospice physician follows the patient in all environments.

Obviously, this includes home visits or house calls. While there is individual variation in frequency of home visits among Hospices, the reassurance that such service is available helps the patient feel comfortable about remaining in the home environment. Physician availability for home visits reaffirms the belief of Hospice patients that they are not being abandoned by the attending physician. In fact, they often receive more direct medical care than that provided by traditional medicine.

It is important to note that more physicians are becoming full-time Hospice medical directors, which enables them to provide more direct, hands-on care to terminally ill patients. The role of this specialist physician is not to supplant the primary care physician. The primary care physician is encouraged to use the palliative care specialist Hospice physician as a consultant. Often in rural areas this is the model that applies, with the primary physician making the house calls.

The role of the Hospice medical director, includes quality assurance. (See "What Is Meant by 'Quality Assurance' in the Hospice Program?" in Chapter 1.) This sometimes leads to conflict if the primary care physician refuses to do an adequate job of managing symptoms. It is the duty of the Hospice physician to assure that symptoms are managed, even if it means stepping over the primary care physician to do so. Most patients and their families are in agreement with this approach, since they desire comfort for the patient and are not concerned about which physician provides it.

The attending physician working with a Hospice is allowed to define his or her role in continuing to care for the patient. For some physicians, this means continuing to care for the patient without any assistance from the Hospice medical director.

More commonly, however, the primary attending physician decides to remain as primary physician with the Hospice medical director serving as a consultant in pain and symptom management. This shared responsibility works best, since the patient is able to continue an already established relationship with the primary care (attending) physician while benefiting from the expertise of the Hospice medical director in pain and symptom control.

The patient is never forced to change physicians; however, more and more physicians are making direct referrals to Hospice physicians for management. This is particularly true when geographic obstacles—primarily distance— interfere with the primary attending physician's ability to visit the now-homebound patient. This is the primary reason that physicians relinquish care to the Hospice medical director.

Even after referral of a patient to the Hospice medical director, it is essential for the Hospice physician to maintain contact with the primary attending physician, to reassure the patient and family that the former physician is aware of current problems and care.

The establishment of strong positive working relationships between primary attending and Hospice physicians is the ultimate answer to the question, "Who is my doctor?" By working together with the Hospice interdisciplinary team, both physicians can provide essential services to the patient and family unit of care. Communication is the key to this successful working relationship, with the Hospice physician being responsible for educating the primary attending physician about the techniques of good palliative medicine.

Together these physicians can provide excellent palliative care for dying patients, their families, and significant others.

Q: How does the patient's attending physician feel about giving a six-month prognosis for the Medicare certified Hospice program? How does the attending physician feel about referring a patient to Hospice? Why do some physicians wait until the death of the patient is imminent before referring the patient to Hospice?

It is often very difficult for physicians to give patients they have cared for and about for a significant length of time an accurate prognosis that they are going to die within the next six months. Many physicians have a great deal of difficulty accepting that their patients are going to die despite their best efforts to cure and save them. This often translates into a reluctance to refer their patients for Hospice care until the last possible moment, resulting in a referral that comes too late for the Hospice to be effective in palliating symptoms and helping the patient and his or her family prepare for death.

Some physicians see making a Hospice referral as a defeat. They may be afraid that their patients may give up hope and succumb to their disease earlier than they would without the Hospice referral. Others are unable to stop aggressive treatment if the slightest chance of improvement remains, even at the expense of debilitating side effects from a last-ditch round of chemotherapy or other treatment.

Michael E. Frederich, M.D., recognized the reluctance of some physicians to accept the death of their patients, specifically identifying discomfort with death as the fifth stumbling block (Frederich, 1991). Orville Moody identified this as well:

Some years ago . . . I organized a conference for other doctors on death. The attendance was much smaller than I had anticipated, and many of those that were present were reluctant to speak up. Doctors seem to fear death intensely, maybe that's why they became doctors (Moody, 1975).

Discomfort with death unfortunately prevents some physicians from ever making a Hospice referral. It is an ethical dilemma for them and, as such, should be handled appropriately, like other dilemmas. A physician unwilling to make a necessary referral, should ask the assistance of a colleague if unable to help his or her patients in this most trying time of their lives. In this way, the patient will receive appropriate palliative care while the physician avoids an uncomfortable situation.

The long-term solution to this problem, however, is education. By including death and dying information in their required curricula, medical schools are beginning to help physicians view death as a normal stage of life: something to be dealt with rationally and not feared and avoided irrationally.

References

Frederich, M. E., "Five Stumbling Blocks to Effective Care for the Terminally Ill," *Hospice Update* (July 1991), 2(3):9-10.

Moody, O., *Make Today Count* (New York: Lippincott, 1975).

Q: Does Hospice force religion or spirituality on its patients?

No. Hospice reaffirms the human spirit. Hospice does not advocate any particular religion or spiritual entity, but most workers in Hospice care embrace the concept that every human being has a spirit that requires nurturing. This philosophy of spirituality includes patients who practice a particular religion and those who consider themselves atheists or agnostics.

In freeing the human spirit from suffering by excellent pain and symptom management, the Hospice team enables the patient and family to redirect energy toward maintaining and nurturing relationships.

Hospice pastoral care and clergy consultants, while sometimes directly serving patients and families to meet their spiritual needs, more often contact the patient's own clergy to make them aware of the patient's situation so the clergy can meet the spiritual needs of the patient and family.

> The spirit is an entity that enables us to maintain our integrity, holding ourselves together when we feel like we are falling apart. It allows us to transcend problems and events beyond our control that threaten to destroy us, and helps us relate to the spirit of other human beings and to higher powers (Erb, 1992).

By reaffirming and supporting the human spirit, Hospice meets the needs of our patients and families in all dimensions. Balfour Mount, M.D., Director of Palliative Care at the Royal Victoria Hospital in Montreal, was asked, "Why do we as physicians and nurses provide pastoral or spirit care?" His answer is, "The spirit dimension is relational; it affects symptoms. Needs of the spirit focus care. If not me or us, who? It will make us effective as team players and we are accepted and chosen by the patient to give it" (Mount, 1990).

Hospice helps provide care for the human spirit while caring for the physical, psychosocial, and other needs of patients and their families.

References

Erb, Art, Personal communication, August 1992.

Mount, Balfour, "Beyond Physical and Psychosocial Care," Estes Park, CO: Keynote Presentation, Sixth International Hospice Institute Symposium, July 22, 1990.

See also "How Will the Spiritual Needs of the Patients, Families, and Significant Others Be Met by the Hospice Program?" in Chapter 1.

Q: What is the importance of symptom relief in terminal care?

Symptom relief is the single most important part of the care that Hospice provides. If we are unable to keep the patient comfortable and relieved from such horrible symptoms as continuous nausea and vomiting, there is no possibility the patient will be able to deal with problems of a financial, psychosocial, or spiritual nature. When an individual is dying, there is an incredible amount of work to be done. If symptoms are not controlled, this work cannot be accomplished and the patient is at risk of dying with unfinished business. (See "What Is 'Unfinished Business'?" in Chapter 1.)

In managing symptoms, a very well organized approach has been outlined by Gary Johanson, M.D., Medical Director of Hospice of Sonoma County, California:

> First, there must be clearly defined medical leadership with an agreement between attending and hospice physicians about division of responsibilities. Next, assessment is crucial with specific attention to a symptom inquiry (defining the source of symptoms), and physical examination followed by specific and limited diagnostic testing. A determination is then made whether this symptom represents basic disease, treatment side-effect, a new illness or just general weakness and debility.
>
> Once the diagnostic impression is formed, communication with the patient and family must occur to explain mechanisms involved and to discuss treatment options and strategy. Medications are prescribed prophylactically (to prevent symptoms from occurring) and simply, attempting to find one medication to serve two functions. Unnecessary medications are discontinued.
>
> Finally, advice is always to be sought and accepted from expert colleagues, explicit instructions are given to all parties involved including hospice staff, patient, and family, and the patient is reassessed often, particularly to assure he or she is compliant with the treatment plan (Johanson, 1990).

Only with such attention to detail can symptoms be adequately managed.

Often in controlling symptoms in the home, nontraditional medications are used. Particularly in the area of managing nausea and vomiting, management may include the prescription of haloperidol, scopolamine, or cannabis (marijuana). Each of these medications is not experimental and has been prescribed effectively in controlling these often difficult symptoms. Also, combinations of medications have been used that might be viewed as unwanted polypharmacy if used for other patients. Hospice has indeed often brought new knowledge and skills regarding management of symptoms to traditional medicine and has helped improve symptom control and palliative care for nonterminal patients.

Reference

Johanson, G. A., "Control of Non-pain Symptoms," Estes Park, CO: Sixth International Hospice Institute Symposium, July 19, 1990.

Q: How can the physical pain of a terminally ill patient be adequately alleviated?

Oddly enough, the answer to this question is "fairly easily." Most physical pain can be alleviated. Using techniques developed and perfected by Hospices, most pain is effectively managed in the patient's home with oral medication.

The first step in managing pain is doing a thorough assessment and teaching the patient to use a communication tool to express adequately the level of pain experienced. A modified McGill scale (Melzack, 1975) using levels one to five, with one being little pain and five the most intense pain imaginable, works well instead of vague descriptions such as "hurting," "shooting," "burning," etc.

The World Health Organization has developed a three-step approach to cancer pain management (World Health Organization, 1986). The first step is using an anti-inflammatory medication to combat pain caused by inflammation and neurostimulating substances produced by the tumor. The second step involves using weak opioid medications such as codeine, oxycodone, and hydrocodone on a routine basis around-the-clock, to control pain completely. By saturating opioid receptors in the brain, both step-two weak opioids and step-three strong opioids keep the patient in a state of comfort. When step-three strong opioids are indicated, most often morphine is prescribed as the drug of choice. It is most often prescribed orally in sustained-release and immediate release forms. The sustained-release form is effective for eight to twelve hours and helps maintain a steady state level of morphine for patient comfort. The immediate-release form can be taken every hour or two as needed for breakthrough pain not controlled by the sustained-release dose.

A fourth step involves treating neuropathic pain or pain caused by direct damage to nerves. This pain is often described as shooting or burning and sometimes becomes so severe that patients cannot stand anything, including clothing, touching their skin. This type of pain does not respond to opioids such as morphine and must be treated with other medication. Fortunately, this pain does respond to antiseizure and antidepressant medications such as sodium valproate, nortriptyline, and carbamazepine.

Even when the patient is unable to take oral medications, he or she can remain comfortable at home. Many of these medications can be administered rectally or under the patient's tongue. If neither of these routes is available, intravenous administration or subcutaneous administration is possible at home.

Patient choice also plays a role in the management of pain in Hospice patients. Some patients may choose to have pain at a very low level of discomfort (level one or two) in order to maintain function, while others may choose to have pain completely relieved and may accept sedation as a side-effect of complete relief. The patient rightfully remains in control of this decision regarding care as long as is possible and practical. Competent, expert management is available for pain control and symptom management in a Hospice program.

References

Foley, K. M., "The Treatment of Cancer Pain," *New England Journal of Medicine* (1985), 313:84-95.

Melzack, R.,"The McGill Pain Questionnaire: Major Properties and Scoring Methods," *Pain* (1975), 1:277.

World Health Organization, *Cancer Pain Relief* (Geneva: World Health Organization, 1986).

Q: Will I become addicted to narcotics if I take them for pain? Will they hasten the end? Does Hospice use too much morphine?

Most studies done to evaluate addiction from narcotics were originally done on people who were already addicts. None of these individuals had pain.

Pain is the best prevention against addiction. If addiction is defined as a psychological dependence and craving for narcotics, it does not happen in people with pain.

Neither are narcotics poisonous; they do not damage specific organs. Although in the past most physicians prescribing narcotics have feared respiratory depression, recent work by Bruera and colleagues (Bruera et al., 1990) has shown that judicious use of opioids can improve respiration rather than impair it.

Rather than hastening death, narcotics such as morphine result in improvement in function and increased quality time due to adequate pain control. Improvement can be very dramatic, with patients previously confined to bed by pain for months being able to resume normal activities such as puttering in the garage, going fishing, and playing with grandchildren after the pain is adequately controlled.

Hospice does not use too much morphine. Often the total dose required for comfort, when given routinely, is less than that required when given on an "as needed" basis. Less medication is needed when pain is controlled, and pain relief is not being "chased ineffectively" by smaller inadequate doses given more often that do not get ahead of the pain and stop it. Instead, by dosing morphine routinely around the clock, it is possible to saturate the brain's morphine receptors and assure continuing pain relief.

In fact, once pain is completely controlled, most Hospice programs advocate slightly decreasing the total dose of morphine administered. Enabling patients to function comfortably at their full potential is the true goal of every Hospice program.

Reference

Bruera, Eduardo, et al., "Effects of Morphine on the Dyspnea of Terminal Cancer Patients," *Journal of Pain and Symptom Management* (December 1990), 5(6):341-4.

Q: How does the Hospice physician feel about honoring patient and family requests concerning "patient self-determination": the health care proxy, do-not-resuscitate orders, living wills, and the durable power of attorney?

In general, Hospice physicians have been some of the strongest advocates among medical professionals for patient autonomy. Because each of the entities (living will, durable power of attorney, etc.) relies on patient autonomy as the foundation principle in medical ethics (Areen, 1987; Greco, 1991; O'Rourke, 1991), most Hospice physicians have no problem honoring these directives.

As always, there are exceptions, particularly if cultural beliefs interfere. For instance, in some cultures withholding food and water is never accepted, and some Hospice physicians may have problems honoring these directives if the patient's durable power of attorney insists that the patient in a chronic vegetative state be given no artificial hydration (Ahronheim and Gasner, 1990; Lo and Dornbrand, 1989). In this instance, it would be the prerogative of the durable power of attorney to seek another physician.

In most cases, however, Hospice physicians are happy to support advance directives in any form because they guide decisions, even if the patient becomes incompetent to continue guiding his or her own plan of care. Direction is helpful, especially in avoiding legal entanglements that have the potential for interfering with the competent medical management of pain and symptoms in the terminally ill. When there is a conflict between physician and family, it is best to try to mediate them within the medical system rather than resort to the courts. Court battles concerning patients such as Nancy Cruzan have led to situations in which medical and/or ethical issues have been decided by the courts or legislature and tend to inhibit the patient-physician and family-physician relationship (Charnow, 1990).

References

Ahronheim, J. C., and M. R. Gasner, "Viewpoint: The Sloganism of Starvation," *Lancet* (1990), 1(335):278-9.

Areen, J., "The Legal Status of Consent Obtained from Families of Adult Patients to Withhold or Withdraw Treatment," *Journal of the American Medical Association* (1987), 258(2):229-35.

Charnow, J. A., "Cruzan Decision Puts Physicians on the Line in Discussing Options," *American College of Physicians Magazine* (1990), 10(8):5-7.

Greco, P. J., K. A. Schulman, R. Lavizzo-Moury, and J. Hansen-Flaschen, "The Patient Self-Determination Act and the Future of Advance Directives," *Annals of Internal Medicine* (1991), 115:639-43.

Lo, B., and L. Dornbrand, "Understanding the Benefits and Burdens of Tube Feedings," *Arch Intern Med* (1989), 149:1925-6.

O'Rourke, K., "Coming Soon to Your Neighborhood Health Care Facility: The Patient Self-Determination Act," *Ethical Issues in Health Care* (St. Louis, MO: Center for Health Care Ethics, St. Louis University Medical Center, May 1991), 12(9):1-2.

Q: What happens at the time of the patient's death in a Hospice program?

Metaphysically, it is difficult to answer this question. Physically, most of the time death for the Hospice patient is quiet, peaceful, and not dramatic. There usually is no increased suffering or pain immediately prior to the cessation of breathing and heart function. Literally, most Hospice patients just sleep away.

There is no attempt at resuscitation of Hospice patients because such efforts will not be beneficial in most instances and would only prolong suffering. Occasionally family members panic at the time of death and call 911. Most Hospice programs attempt to avoid this last-minute confusion by having do-not-resuscitate orders, living wills, and other forms of advance directives for most patients. Nurses of Hospice of Southern Illinois, Inc., have been trained to tell patients and their families that they are their "911 service" and to call them first in the event of any emergency. This has avoided much confusion and unnecessary turmoil and distress for the patient and family.

Most Hospice programs respond to death by sending the nurse out to the home. Helping the family with acute bereavement and grief problems is paramount. In addition, the nurse facilitates the process of notification of appropriate resources, including the coroner and funeral home.

The bereavement support of the surviving family member(s) actively begins at this time (Brown, 1992). Also, the bereavement and grief work of Hospice personnel is helped by their attendance at the funeral to say good-bye to the patient they have come to love over the days, weeks, and months of care in the Hospice program. Usually bereavement follow-up continues for family members for a period of at least twelve months, often longer if abnormal grief occurs.

By identifying risk factors for abnormal grief and maintaining close ties to the family, the bereavement counselor can become more involved if abnormal grief occurs or refer the family to resources outside Hospice for greater depth or psychological counseling and support. Many Hospices also maintain grief support groups or use community-based resources such as Widow to Widow groups for support of grieving family members.

References

Brown, W. W., "When My Patient Dies" and "Caring for the Bereaved," in *Death and Dying: Working with the Life-Threatened Patient and Family* (St. Louis, MO: St. Louis University School of Medicine, 1992), 276-306; 307-50.

See also "Bereavement," Chapter 11.

See also "What Happens When a Patient Dies at Home? What Does the Family Do?" in Chapter 2.

9
MEDICARE HOSPICE BENEFITS

1. What are the Medicare Hospice benefits? Who can provide them?

2. What is the difference between the Hospice benefit and other Medicare benefits?

3. Who is eligible to receive Medicare Hospice benefits? How is payment made for these benefits? How long can Hospice care continue? Where can I get more information about the Medicare program?

4. Are there special Medicare requirements for a certified Hospice program?

5. What are the pertinent Medicare Hospice definitions and the levels of Hospice reimbursement?

6. Does the Medicare Hospice benefit cover the cost of this care? What about other third-party payors?

7. What is the interdisciplinary team (IDT)?

8. The interdisciplinary team (IDT): What is the involvement of the patient, family members, and significant others?

9. What else is required of the interdisciplinary team (IDT) and other Hospice staff, in addition to providing their professional expertise?

10. What are *core services* and *contracted services* in a Medicare certified Hospice program? Who is responsible for coordinating, contracting for, and monitoring these services?

11. What is the "Patient/Family Plan of Care"?

12. Can people with end-stage Alzheimer's Disease and their families be helped in a Medicare certified Hospice program?

13. What is Hospice day care?

14. What is meant by "drugs and biologicals" in a Medicare certified Hospice program?

15. What is the difference between a Hospice and a regular home health agency?

16. What is the difference between a Medicare Hospice program and a palliative care program?

Q: What are the Medicare Hospice benefits? Who can provide them?

Medicare Hospice benefits can be provided only by a Medicare certified Hospice program that has met *all* the requirements and been approved by the Health Care Financing Administration of the United States Department of Health and Human Services. The program also must pass periodic surveys conducted by the Department of Health, meet the individual state and local requirements, and receive an "operating certificate" that is renewed periodically after additional surveys.

Hospice care can be provided by a public agency or organization that is primarily engaged in furnishing services to terminally ill individuals and their families. To receive Medicare payment, the agency or organization must be certified by Medicare to provide Hospice services.

[Medicare Hospice] certification is required even if the agency or organization is already approved by Medicare to provide other kinds of health services. Patients can find out whether a Hospice program is certified by Medicare by asking their physician or checking with the agency or organization offering the program (*Medicare Hospice Benefits*).

(See Appendix A, Figure 10, "Organizational Chart by Employment and Supervision" for an independent, community-based, not-for-profit Hospice program.)

There are special rules that govern Medicare's coverage of, and payment for, Hospice care. The Health Care Financing Administration (HCFA) defines Hospice care as

. . . a special way of caring for a patient whose disease cannot be cured. It is available as a benefit under Medicare Hospital Insurance (Part A). Medicare beneficiaries who choose to have Hospice care receive a full scope of non-curative medical and support services for their terminal illness while continuing to live in their own homes. They must be certified by a physician to be terminally ill with a life expectancy of about six months or less. They no longer receive treatment toward a cure, but require close medical and supportive care. (See also "What Are the Pertinent Medicare Definitions and the Levels of Hospice Reimbursement?" in this chapter.)

What Are Medicare's Hospice Benefits?

Under Medicare, Hospice is primarily a comprehensive home care program that provides all the reasonable and necessary medical and support services for the management of a terminal illness. Medicare covers:

- Physician services
- Nursing care
- Medical appliances and supplies
- Outpatient drugs for symptom management and pain relief
- Short-term respite care in an inpatient setting, to provide respite for a family or others caring for the individual at home (limited to five days)
- Short-term care in an inpatient setting for pain control or acute or chronic symptom management
- Home health aide and homemaker services
- Audiology, physical therapy, occupational therapy, respiratory therapy, and speech/language pathology services
- Medical social services
- Nutrition and dietary counseling
- Anticipatory grief and bereavement counseling, and
- Other supportive counseling services as needed—psychological, spiritual, pastoral, legal, financial, etc.

When a patient receives these services from a Medicare certified Hospice, Medicare hospital insurance pays almost the entire cost. The only expense to the beneficiary is limited cost-sharing for outpatient drugs and inpatient respite care.

Are Other Medicare Benefits Available in Addition to Hospice Care?

When Medicare beneficiaries choose Hospice care, they give up the right to standard Medicare benefits for treatment of the terminal illness. Medicare pays the entire cost of the covered services required to manage the illness, except the co-payments for respite care and outpatient prescription drugs and biologicals. A Hospice patient can, however, qualify for standard Medicare benefits if:

- The patient requires covered Medicare services for the treatment of a condition *unrelated* to the terminal illness.
- The patient has Medicare Medical Insurance (Part B) and the patient's attending physician is not working for the Hospice. In that case, Medicare Part B will help pay for the physician's services. Medicare pays 80 percent of the approved amount for covered services after the patient meets the Part B annual deductible ($100 in 1996).

What Is Not Covered?

Hospice coverage is in effect only for conditions related to the individual patient's terminal illness.

All services for treatment of the terminal illness must be provided by or through the Hospice. When a Medicare beneficiary chooses Hospice care, Medicare will *not* pay for:

- Treatment for the terminal illness that is not for symptom management and pain control
- Treatment for an injury or other illness not related to the terminal condition
- Care provided by another Hospice that was not arranged by the patient's Hospice
- Care from another provider that duplicates care the Hospice is required to provide.

Note that Medicare certified Hospices have contractual arrangements with one or more hospitals or nursing homes. Usually, the patient's primary physician either is on the contracted hospital/nursing home staff or has staff privileges arranged by the

Hospice. However, if this is not so, or if it is not the hospital or nursing home of choice for some other reason, the patient/family may consider choosing a different Hospice program.

An example of treatment and care in a situation *not* related to the terminal illness follows. The patient may fall, break a leg, and require hospitalization to have the leg set. In this situation, regular (non-Hospice) Medicare coverage—and other insurance, if applicable—provide(s) coverage. This does *not* affect the Medicare Hospice coverage. The Hospice still is responsible for overseeing the care of this patient and works with the patient's physician to make arrangements and specify all details in the individual patient's plan of care.

Reference

Medicare Hospice Benefits, U.S. Department of Health and Human Services: Health Care Financing Administration (HCFA), Publication No. HCFA 386-894/00507, 1995.

Q: What is the difference between the Hospice benefit and other Medicare benefits?

The primary difference between the Hospice Medicare benefit and other Medicare benefits is in the support system that is available, not just to the patient, but also to the family and significant others. In the Hospice program, home health care is primary and available, even if the patient is not homebound, confined to bed, or in need of skilled nursing care at the time of admission. Care is provided even if the patient has not just been discharged from the hospital.

"The hospice benefit under Medicare is designed to be more than just a collection of existing benefits with a new name. Many items and services are covered under hospice that are not covered through any other type of facility or provider" (*Hospice Benefit,* 1992).

The New York State Hospice Association has designed a chart to show a comparison of Medicare benefits available through three types of Medicare certified providers: a qualified Hospice, a hospital, and a home health agency. (See Appendix A, Figure 11.)

Note: Under "Service/Items," there are no deductibles and no co-insurance is required, with the exception of a 5 percent co-payment for medications and respite care (*Hospice Benefit,* 1992).

Reference

The Hospice Benefit and Other Medicare Benefits (White Plains, NY: New York State Hospice Association, January 1992).

Q: Who is eligible to receive Medicare Hospice benefits?

Hospice care is available only if:

- The patient is eligible for Medicare Hospital Insurance (Part A)
- The patient's doctor and the Hospice medical director certify that the patient is terminally ill
- The patient signs a statement choosing Hospice care instead of standard Medicare benefits for the terminal illness
- The patient receives care from a Medicare certified Hospice program (*Medicare Hospice Benefits*).

Any patient with terminal illness is a candidate for Hospice care. The majority of people cared for by Hospice have cancer, but patients with end-stage chronic diseases such as congestive heart failure, chronic obstructive pulmonary disease, cystic fibrosis, Alzheimer's Disease, renal failure, and AIDS have been Hospice patients. (See Appendix A, Figure 12, "Medicare Hospice Benefits Election.")

How Is Payment Made for These Benefits?

Medicare pays the Hospice directly at specified rates, depending on the type of care given each day. The patient is responsible only for:

- *Drugs or biologicals:* The Hospice can charge 5 percent of the reasonable cost, up to a maximum of $5, for each prescription for outpatient drugs or biologicals for pain relief and symptom management. (See "What Is Meant by 'Drugs and Biologicals' in a Medicare Certified Hospice Program?" in this chapter.)

- *Respite care:* The Hospice may periodically arrange for inpatient care for the patient to give temporary relief to the person who regularly provides care in the home. Respite care is limited each time to a stay of no more than 5 days. The patient can be charged about $4 per day for respite care. The charge varies slightly, depending on the geographic area of the country (*Medicare Hospice Benefits*).

(See "What Are the Pertinent Medicare Definitions and the Levels of Hospice Reimbursement?" in this chapter.)

How Long Can Hospice Care Continue?

Special benefit periods apply to Hospice care. A patient can receive Medicare-covered Hospice care as long as a physician certifies that the patient is terminally ill. A Medicare beneficiary can choose to receive Hospice care for two 90-day benefit periods, followed by a 30-day period, that can, when necessary, be extended indefinitely [into a fourth benefit period]. The periods may be used consecutively or at intervals. Regardless of whether they are used one right after the other or at different times, the patient must be certified as terminally ill at the beginning of each period [by the patient's attending physician and the Hospice medical director].

A patient who chooses Hospice care may change Hospice programs once [in] each benefit period [without affecting the number of covered days]. A patient also has the right to cancel Hospice care at any time and return to standard Medicare coverage, then later re-elect the Hospice benefit *if* another benefit period is available. If the patient cancels Hospice care during one of the first three benefit periods, any days left in that period are lost, but the patient is still eligible for the remaining benefit period(s). For example, if a patient cancels at the end of 60 days in the first 90-day period, the remaining 30 days in the period are forfeited. The patient is, however, still eligible for the second 90-day period, the 30-day period, and the indefinite extension. If cancellation occurs during the final [indefinite extension] period, the patient *cannot* use the Hospice benefit again, [ever].

(See Appendix A, Figure 13, "Hospice Benefit Revocation Form," and Figure 14, "Request for Change of Designated Hospice.")

Where Can I Get More Information About the Medicare Program?

For more information about the Medicare program, please refer to *The Medicare Handbook.* Any Social Security Office has free copies available.

Reference

Medicare Hospice Benefits, U.S. Department of Health and Human Services: Health Care Financing Administration (HCFA), Publication No. HCFA 386-894/00507, 1995.

Q: Are there special Medicare requirements for a certified Hospice program?

There are some special services Medicare requires of all participating certified Hospice programs. These cover *periods of crisis, respite care, bereavement counseling,* and *volunteer services.*

- *Periods of crisis:* Nursing care may be covered on a continuous basis for as much as 24 hours per day during periods of crisis. Either homemaker or home health aide services or both may be covered on a 24-hour continuous basis during periods of crisis, but care during these periods must be predominantly nursing care—to achieve palliation or management of acute medical symptoms.
- *Respite care:* Respite care may be provided on an occasional basis and may not be reimbursed for more than five consecutive days at a time.
- *Bereavement counseling:* Bereavement counseling services are a required Hospice service provided to the individual's family for up to one year after the individual's death. However, it is *not* reimbursable by Medicare.
- *Volunteer services:* At least 5 percent of total Hospice hours must be provided by specially trained volunteers. In addition to providing office back-up and support, "Good Neighbor" volunteers help patients, families, and significant

others in a variety of ways, including visiting, child care, tutoring, shopping, transportation, providing caring, compassionate listening, and practical support. (There is no reimbursement for the volunteer program. Hospices must raise funds to provide skilled training, supervision, and the required ongoing support and services for their volunteer programs.)

Q: What are the pertinent Medicare Hospice definitions and the levels of Hospice reimbursement?

For clarity and understanding, it is important to define pertinent Hospice Medicare terminology, including the four levels of care.

- *Periods of crisis:* A period in which the individual requires continuous care, which is primarily nursing care, to achieve palliation or management of acute medical symptoms.
- *Representative:* A person who is, because of the individual's mental or physical incapacity, authorized in accordance with state law to execute or revoke an election for Hospice care or terminate medical care on behalf of the terminally ill individual.
- *Election period:* One of four periods for which an individual may elect to receive Medicare coverage of Hospice care. The periods consist of (consecutively) two 90-day periods, one 30-day period, and a fourth, indefinite, period.
- *Free-Standing hospice:* A Hospice that is not part of any other type of participating provider.

Levels of Care

Medicare reimburses certified Hospice programs directly, on a *per diem* basis "at specified rates depending on the type of care given each day." There are four levels of care, as described below.

The rate of reimbursement is adjusted annually by the Health Care Financing Administration (HCFA). This is a cost-of-living adjustment (COLA) and varies for each program, depending upon demographics and where the Hospice is located in the United States.

1. *Routine home care day:* A day on which an individual who has elected to receive Hospice care is at home and not receiving continuous home care that is predominantly nursing care. A routine home care day could include respite care delivered in the home.

2. *Continuous home care day:* A day on which an individual who has elected to receive Hospice care is not in an inpatient facility and receives Hospice care, predominantly nursing care, on a continuous basis at home during periods of crisis for a duration of at least 8 hours.

3. *Inpatient respite care day:* A day on which the individual who has elected Hospice care receives care only when necessary to relieve the family members (or other persons caring for the individual at home) on a short-term basis in an approved inpatient facility, for not more than five days.

4. *General inpatient care day:* A day on which an individual who has elected to receive Hospice care receives general inpatient care in an inpatient facility for pain control or acute or chronic symptom management that cannot be managed in other settings.

References

Code of Federal Regulations: Public Health 42 Part 418: Hospice Care, Washington, DC 42 C.F.R. chapter IV (10/1/86 Edition, approved 2/10/87), Part 418.302: Hospice Reimbursement Methods (Categories).

Medicare Hospice Benefits, U.S. Department of Health and Human Services: Health Care Financing Administration (HCFA), Publication No. HCFA 386-894/00507, 1995.

Q: Does the Medicare Hospice Benefit cover the cost of this care? What about other third-party payors?

Although Medicare pays Hospice directly for the services provided, payments are less than what it actually costs Hospice programs to provide the Medicare-mandated services to patients, their families, and significant others.

For non-Medicare-eligible patients, Hospice programs receive other reimbursement for services provided to Medicaid-eligible patients/families, those who have private insurance coverage, including coverage from health maintenance organizations (HMOs), perhaps by contractual arrangement with the individual Hospice program. Some patients and families are charged fees for services, according to their ability to pay, when insurance coverage either does not exist or provides inadequate reimbursement. (See also Chapter 1, "Who Pays for the Services Provided by Hospice Programs?")

No patient/family is refused service because of the nature of the disease, race, sex, age, religion, or inability to pay. Many Hospice programs provide special outreach to the indigent and the underserved.

In all of these cases, payments to Hospices continue to be less than the cost of services provided. Frequently, the financial shortfall may range from 25 to 30 percent each year.

For survival of the Hospice programs, this inadequate reimbursement must be made up by generous contributions and active community involvement. Donations of dollars, time, and in-kind services, bequests and memorial contributions, government, corporate, and foundation grants, and proceeds from various fundraising projects all are inspirational examples of communities that care about their people and work together to make it possible for Hospice programs to survive, enabling them to serve the communities that support them.

Q: What is the interdisciplinary team (IDT)?

The interdisciplinary team (IDT) is the entity created to provide and coordinate Hospice services to the patient/family unit. The focus is to help the patient remain at home.

Team clinical skills help monitor pain control and symptom management to keep the patient as alert and comfortable as possible. Team members also support and teach the family and significant others how to care for the patient at home and for themselves. The team provides whatever supportive services are necessary to help cope with the feelings and problems that arise during this difficult time and after the death of the patient.

It is the role of IDT members to be sensitive to the unique needs of the patient/family and significant others, as a group as well as individually. The IDT also provides for relief (respite) for family and caregivers, who may neglect their own needs while caring for the patient (and, perhaps, other family members). (See also "What

Else Is Required of the Interdisciplinary Team (IDT) and Other Hospice Staff?" in this chapter.)

The Hospice IDT consists of physicians (including the patient's attending physician), nurses, medical social workers, nutritionist, pharmacist(s), home health aides, pastoral counselors, and specially trained volunteers—as well as various therapists and experts in other fields who are called upon as needed. Specifically, the team is composed of the following representatives:

1. Medical director
2. Patient care coordinator
3. Social worker(s)
4. Pastoral care coordinator
5. Director of volunteers
6. Core Hospice nurses assigned to case
7. Volunteer(s) assigned to case
8. Nutritionist and other personnel assigned to case.

In addition, the following representatives may choose to participate or may be requested to participate in team meetings, as necessary:

1. Executive director
2. Primary care physician
3. Contract agency personnel assigned to Hospice case
4. Mental health consultant
5. Pharmacy consultant
6. Bereavement coordinator
7. Other medical or professional specialty area representative(s)
8. Attending clergy person.

(See also "What Are *Core* Services and *Contracted* Services in a Medicare Certified Hospice Program?" in this chapter.)

The IDT meets on a regular schedule (which will vary to meet the needs of individual Hospice programs) to prepare, implement, review, and revise each patient/family plan of care. (See "What Is the 'Patient/Family Plan of Care'? in this chapter.)

In addition to the scheduled formal meetings (which are carefully documented), there is also informal contact among IDT members (including trained volunteers) by phone or in informal meetings, as the need arises, to discuss patient/family care and any changes in the situation.

Q: The interdisciplinary team (IDT): What is the involvement of the patient, family members, and significant others?

Patients, family members (including children), and significant others are considered members of the IDT. Ideally, they are kept fully informed and actively involved in decision making, to the degree in which they choose to participate. Hospice services are provided to the patient *and* family as the "unit of care," with the focus of providing care primarily in the home. This team involvement gives the patient/family unit a greater degree of control over what happens during the time that is left—helping to alleviate some feelings of helplessness, frustration, and inadequacy. This also gives the family and significant others the opportunity to maintain a close relationship in familiar surroundings at home and care for their ill loved one and each other under the professional and compassionate guidance of the Hospice IDT.

Q: What else is required of the interdisciplinary team (IDT) and other Hospice staff?

Every member of the Hospice staff works with or for the patient, family, and significant others, either directly or indirectly. This is because the Hospice's only reason for being is to provide comprehensive, compassionate care for those who have a limited life expectancy *and* for their families and significant others.

All staff—whether paid or volunteer, full-time or part-time, professional or nonprofessional, in-house or subcontracted—are part of a total environment of compassionate palliative care for the patient, family, and significant others in the Hospice program. For this reason, each employee and volunteer is "expected to function as part of a team, as well as in the specific areas of competence for which he or she has been hired."

This hospice staff interdependence involves the following essential components for all employees and volunteers:

1. Willingness to attend and participate in team meetings, with a commitment to teamwork, team building, and the achievement of team goals.

2. Willingness to express concern and to care personally for patients, their families, and significant others.

3. Willingness to participate in ongoing staff development and support programs.

4. Willingness to learn new information and methods in care for the dying and their families, including care of AIDS patients and significant others.

5. Willingness to be interested in and supportive to other Hospice staff members.

6. Willingness to work closely with volunteers as fellow staff.

7. Willingness to share in twenty-four (24) hour/day, seven (7) day/week availability, as specified in the terms of employment for each employee.

8. Commitment to quality health care, high professional standards, and respect for the various disciplines represented in Hospice.

9. Respect and concern for the values and desires of patient/families and significant others, whatever their culture, nationality, or religion, and commitment to the Statement of Hospice Patient/Family Rights.

Reference

"Personnel Policies and Procedures: 'General Staff Statement' " (Hempstead, NY: Long Island Foundation for Hospice Care and Research, Inc., 1988), p. 5.

Q: What are *core services* and *contracted services* in a Medicare certified Hospice program? Who is responsible for coordinating, contracting for, and monitoring these services?

Core services are routinely provided directly by Hospice employees. Core services include:

- Direct professional nursing services in the home setting
- Physician services for medical consultation and for the general medical care of patients to the extent that such needs are not met by the patient's own attending physician
- Medical social services

- Counseling—including "anticipatory grief" and bereavement support
- Nutritional/dietary counseling.

Contracted services refer to additional Hospice services, provided by contractual arrangement, by professional providers who are not in the direct employ of the Hospice. These also are Medicare-mandated services to be provided as and when needed as part of the palliation/comfort care for the terminal illness. Contracted services include:

- Physical therapy
- Occupational therapy
- Respiratory therapy
- Speech/language pathology
- Audiology
- Continuous care nursing
- Durable medical equipment, supplies, and appliances
- Psychological/psychiatric services
- Laboratory services
- Pharmaceutical services
- General inpatient care
- Respite inpatient care
- Home health aides
- Personal care aides
- Homemakers/housekeepers
- Ambulance/ambulette transportation services
- And other specialized services that may be needed, such as legal and financial guidance.

The *executive director/administrator* is responsible for negotiating and executing all contracts, with approval and ratification by the governing board of trustees.

The *patient care [nurse] coordinator* is responsible for coordinating and integrating all contracted services into the Hospice program for each patient and family, as specified in the [individualized] Hospice plan of care for each patient/family/significant other(s).

All core services, as well as contracted services by outside providers of care, are under the professional management of Hospice. All staff (including volunteers) take part in an ongoing self-assessment of the appropriateness and quality of the care provided.

An appointed *quality assurance committee* assists the governing board of trustees in its "legal responsibility for determining, implementing and monitoring policies [and services provided] governing the Hospice's total operation." (See also "What Is Meant by 'Quality Assurance' in the Hospice Program?" in Chapter 1.)

References

Certificate of Need (CON) Application to the Department of Health, New York State, for the Establishment of a Certified Hospice Program (Hempstead, NY: Long Island Foundation for Hospice Care and Research, Inc., 1987).

Hospice Operations Manual (Hempstead, NY: Long Island Foundation for Hospice Care and Research, Inc., 1989).

Q: What is the "Patient/Family Plan of Care"?

When a patient is admitted into the Hospice program, a written plan is created and maintained, indicating the services to be provided for each individual. Since the patient/family/significant others are the "unit of care" in a Hospice program, this *patient/family plan of care* specifies the services required ". . . to meet the needs of individuals for care that is reasonable and necessary for the palliation and management of terminal illness and related conditions . . . " (*Hospice Operations Manual*, 1989).

Preparation

The *initial plan of care* is prepared on or before the provision of services to newly admitted patient/families. Usually, it is the admissions nurse who consults with one or more team members. The patient's attending physician also participates in the establishment of the plan of care, and works with the Hospice interdisciplinary team in caring for the patient.

The IDT members meet within 48 hours after these services begin, to develop the *comprehensive plan of care*. This is finalized in written form, approved, signed by the Hospice medical director, and a copy is sent to the attending physician.

Content of Patient/Family Plan of Care

Included in the individual patient's Hospice plan of care are the following:

1. Assessment of the needs of the patient, the family, and significant others
2. Listing of the patient's and family's wants and needs, including any discomfort and symptoms of the patient as a result of the terminal condition
3. All services required to meet patient and family identified needs, specified as to frequency and scope
4. Designation of person(s) taking responsibility for provision of specific services. (Includes team members, family caregivers, and any contracted providers.)

Education and Training

Education and training of the patient, family, and significant others are part of the plan of care. In addition to encouraging the patient, family, and significant others to actively involve themselves in the care planning process, they also are encouraged to participate in the treatment process. Education and training are offered to them on what is happening, what is likely to happen, the processes of dying and grieving, and how they can participate in the implementation of the comprehensive plan of care. Particular emphasis is placed on comfort measures that can be employed.

Implementation

The responsibility for coordinating all contract and direct services and assuring the quality of all contract and direct services rests with the core interdisciplinary team. A periodic team review of patient care services is made. Each department is responsible for implementing its own services, as specified in the plan of care. Overall coordination is the responsibility of the patient care (nurse) coordinator. Continuity within assignment of Hospice staff is maintained as much as possible.

The patient/family/significant others also participate (to the extent with which they feel comfortable)

- In the assessment process, to help identify the problems and services needed
- In discussion(s) of the care plan with the appropriate designated Hospice representative after the plan is formulated
- In discussions of modifications in the care plan as situations change during the Hospice stay.

Review and Revision

Once it is approved and implemented, the Hospice plan of care *can* be changed. This change will reflect the difference, intensity, and level of care needed by the patient, family, and significant others, as their situation follows the course of the terminal illness.

The Hospice plan of care for each patient is reviewed by the interdisciplinary team at least every two weeks (or as needed), with any updated information and care plan revision documented and dated. The plan of care includes the next review date, which will be specific to patient/family needs. This review and update involves

1. The attending physician
2. The Hospice medical director or physician designee
3. The interdisciplinary team, including volunteers
4. Input from patient/family/significant others, as appropriate.

All consultations, meetings (formal and informal), phone contacts, family visits, correspondence, and volunteer contacts, are carefully recorded and documented in the patient/family medical records.

References

Hospice Operations Manual (Hempstead, NY: Long Island Foundation for Hospice Care and Research, Inc., 1989).

Hospice Operations Manual (Ithaca, NY: Hospicare of Thompkins County, 1987).

Q: Can people with end-stage Alzheimer's Disease and their families be helped in a Medicare certified Hospice program?

Yes, people with end-stage Alzheimer's Disease and their families *can* be helped in a Hospice program.

"Alzheimer's Disease is a progressive, degenerative disease that attacks the brain and results in impaired memory, thinking, and behavior." Alzheimer's sufferers eventually become totally incapable of caring for themselves.

Although no cure for Alzheimer's Disease is available at present, good planning and medical and social management can ease the burdens on the patient and family....A calm and well-structured environment may help the afflicted person to maintain as much comfort and dignity as possible....Appropriate medication can lessen agitation, anxiety and unpredictable behavior . . . (*Alzheimer's Disease Fact Sheet*).

As the most common form of dementing illness, Alzheimer's afflicts an estimated 4 million American adults. More than 100,000 people die of Alzheimer's Disease annually (*Alzheimer's Disease Fact Sheet*, 1990). Although most patients are over 65, some can be in their 40s and 50s. However, ". . . the number of Alzheimer victims is expected to increase dramatically with the continued growth of the country's older population," according to the Nassau/Suffolk Counties Chapter of the Alzheimer's Association.

. . . demographics of Alzheimer's Disease in the New York City area are compelling, with over 75,000 living cases. The disease occurs in six percent of the general population over 65 years of age, and twenty percent of those 75 and over. . . . By the year 2050 it is estimated that over fourteen million persons in the United States over age 65 will have Alzheimer's Disease. On the average, somewhere between 60%-70% of residents in nursing homes have some form of dementia (Brenner, 1995).

The same criteria for admission applies to *all* Hospice patients, including those with dementia. Primarily a home care program, Hospice exists to provide palliative comfort care when cure is not possible. The treatment focuses on enhancing comfort for both terminally ill patients *and* their families, and has been proven to be unique and effective.

"Certainly families who have a member with Alzheimer's Disease are stressed by years of caregiving, and could benefit greatly from support, especially as they face the ending of life and want their loved one not to be institutionalized, if that's not necessary" (Brenner, 1995).

An example of this is the *pilot* project and collaborative effort that was started in the fall of 1990 between the Jacob Perlow Hospice, Inc., in Manhattan and the New York City Chapter of the Alzheimer's Association. (The *formal* project, from 1993-1995, was part of the Robert Wood Johnson Local Initiatives Funding Partners Program.)

A summary of the successful pilot project was presented by Jane Weber, then administrator of the Jacob Perlow Hospice, Inc. (September 1991). (Paul Brenner described the total experience in Novermber 1995, with completed documentation and final summary of the project expected in 1996.)

The Program

The Alzheimer's Association will help inform the family members of a patient with dementia about the Hospice choice in terminal care. A referral process has been established to maximize the efficiency of the referral from agency to agency and with the family. The same *admission criteria* applies to a dementia patient as applies to all Hospice patients:

1. A patient diagnosed by a licensed physician as having an advanced disease with a limited life expectancy.
2. A patient under the care of a physician who agrees that Hospice care is appropriate.
3. The patient is a resident of [the Hospice service area] Brooklyn, Queens, or Manhattan.
4. The family consent to Hospice services.
5. The patient had expressed a desire in the past [or the legally designated person, with durable powers of attorney to make health care decisions, decides] that no . . . feeding tube, or other extraordinary treatment occur.
6. A primary careperson in the home is preferred but not required.

The *services* of the interdisciplinary team that provides medical, nursing care, counseling, emotional support, instruction, and practical assistance will be offered both in the home and during short-term stays in the Hospice inpatient unit at Beth Israel [Medical Center]. Every effort will be made to provide aide service by home health aides trained to care for Alzheimer's patients. A member of the Hospice nursing staff is available 24 hours a day, to answer questions, discuss concerns, or handle problems. Follow-up counseling for family members is offered after the patient's death.

The Patient

A referral to Hospice might be indicated if the patient has a combination of the following symptoms or characteristics of a terminally ill Alzheimer patient:

- Profoundly progressed dementia
- Speech ability limited to about half-dozen words
- Intelligible vocabulary limited to a single word
- Ambulatory ability lost
- Ability to sit up lost
- Ability to smile lost
- Ability to hold head up lost
- Difficulty swallowing
- Fecal and urinary incontinence
- Recurrent infections.

Collaboration

Initial educational training was provided by the Alzheimer's Association to the [Jacob Perlow] Hospice staff. A Clinical Advisory Board has been formed to review cases, monitor the program's development, and to affirm or redefine goals for ongoing collaboration. All training sessions are videotaped to provide data for possible research in the future.

One problem is that it may be difficult to place an Alzheimer's patient in a specific stage of the disease. Although symptoms seem to progress in a recognizable pattern (Gwyther, 1985), they are not uniform in all patients and the stages can overlap. "The disease can take anywhere from three to twenty-five years to progress to the advanced stage, and confirmation of diagnosis requires autopsy" (Brenner, 1995).

"Another problem is assessing pain, since Alzheimer's patients cannot describe it—and then determining whether the pain control procedure has worked" (Brenner, 1996).

The long-term nature of this disease leads to another problem. It can be hard to tell when an Alzheimer's patient is in the end-stage of the disease and eligible for Hospice admission. "There was some question as to when an Alzheimer's patient could be certified by a physician as having a prognosis of six months or less," according to Ms. Weber. In a presentation given in 1992, Ms. Weber continued:

> Prognosticators, that have been developed and refined to ascertain when patients are appropriate for Hospice care, are now identifying appropriate patients with Alzheimer's disease for our program. As a result families have been able to care for their loved ones at home throughout the difficult end-stage of the disease. [The Jacob Perlow] Hospice has been able to provide them with the intensive support and services they require, including special therapies during the illness and bereavement care for the family following the patient's death. . . .
>
> It is very clear that Hospice care for Alzheimer's patients greatly reduces the number of days of institutional care allowing patients to remain in their own home (Public Hearings, 1992).

Special education and training must be provided for all Hospice staff as well as for the families and significant others. This is important in helping them

> to understand the demands of caring for Alzheimer's patients; the impact of the length of the illness on the family; the patient's helplessness and "loss of self"; special nursing needs, such as those brought on by feeding difficulties and immobility, and the patient's severe cognitive decline and lack of responsiveness (*Newsletter*, p. 3).

According to Brenner (1995), the Jacob Perlow Hospice experience found that few Hospice volunteers were comfortable working directly with Alzheimer's patients. Most were "involved in providing respite care and support for family members. . . ."

> *Home health aides* provide the most frequently used service by Alzheimer's patients in home care. . . . It is this support that makes the difference in the ability of families to keep a patient at home rather than to seek an institutional placement. . .
>
> *Music therapy* has been used effectively with a number of patients. Since the music response is located in one of the most primitive areas of the brain, there may be a response to music when there is response to little or nothing else. The music therapist carefully researches with the family members songs and tunes that were especially beloved by the patient, usually at an earlier time of life. Music is often connected to specific times of life when life was happy and full. It is also a great comfort to family members [when they] see the patient respond. It is a glimpse of the person they always knew and loved, and that is comforting when rational communication is almost or totally non-existent (Brenner, 1995).

Special project funding was sought to help serve these patients and their families, particularly for the home health aide support at the levels required, and for the services of a music therapist. However—due to the uncertain reimbursement environment and the current levels of Hospice reimbursement (almost exclusively Medicare *and* special funds, the [Jacob Perlow] Hospice established to support uncompensated services)—it is doubtful that the Hospice will be able to continue on that level of support.

> While some families are able to hire private duty aides, most are not. It may be that without supplemental funding, fewer patients may be able to be supported at home and will need nursing home placement (Brenner, 1995).

Family members and significant others have found it extremely difficult to cope with the dementia part of the disease: the loss of memory, patient disorientation, the impaired judgment, and severe deterioration in personality changes. The Hospice team can be there for them 24 hours a day to provide them with compassion, comfort, and solace—and help them live through the trauma of caring for the Alzheimer's patient.

References

Alzheimer's Disease Fact Sheet (Chicago: Alzheimer's Disease and Related Disorders Association, Inc., 1990).

Brenner, Paul R., *The Experience of Jacob Perlow Hospice: Hospice Care of Patients with Alzheimer's Disease* (New York: The Jacob Perlow Hospice, Inc. [A Program of Beth Israel Medical Center], November 1995).

——, Exec. Dir., Jacob Perlow Hospice (New York: Private communication, May 1996).

Gwyther, Lisa P., *Care of Alzheimer's Patients: A Manual for Nursing Home Staff* (Chicago: Alzheimer's Association [Member, Committee on Patient and Family Service], 1985).

Newsletter: The Jacob Perlow Hospice (Summer, 1992), p. 3.

Weber, Jane, *Jacob Perlow Hospice/Alzheimer's Association Project: A Summary* (New York: The Jacob Perlow Hospice, Inc. [A Program of Beth Israel Medical Center], September 1991).

——. "Alzheimer's Disease and Related Disorders," State of New York Joint Public Hearings, November 17, 1992.

Q: What is Hospice day care?

Hospice programs reach out to enhance the quality of life for the patient/family unit of care by creating an atmosphere in which they can experience life as fully as possible. Hospice day care is an extension of the supportive care provided, and evolved out of the recognition, by some Hospices, that there were unmet needs.

A Hospice may operate its own day care facility. Others may contract out these services, perhaps with a nearby hospital or nursing home that has a community outreach program or with a senior citizens' group or local community center.

To meet the individual needs of the patient and family, Hospice day care must be flexible and, ideally, provided in a physical environment that is cheerful, wheelchair accessible, and noninstitutional in decor. Quiet areas and work areas are needed, as is space for various therapies and treatments, including areas for resting, eating, and other activities (Henderson and Holden, 1991).

Hospice day care can include the following:

- Support groups and individual counseling (for patients, their families, and significant others)—an opportunity to share issues and concerns
- Meals in a homelike setting
- Massage therapy and relaxation activities
- Assistance with activities of daily living (ADL)
- Beauty parlor and barber services
- Writers' workshop—creating periodic newsletters about day care activities and people involved
- Music therapy
- Occupational therapy—arts and crafts
- Physical therapy (one day care program provides a whirlpool for patients *and* families)
- Nutrition and diet counseling and cooking classes
- Entertainment, games, and lending library (books, talking books, audiocassettes, and videos)
- Other therapies and medical care that is difficult to access in the home, such as podiatry, audiology, ophthalmology, monitoring medications, medical support, nursing services, dental care, speech/language pathology
- Holiday or birthday celebrations
- Religious services and spiritual support
- Outings and educational programs
- Audiovisual equipment to help patients "tell their story" through autobiographical reminiscences.

Admission Criteria

1. Patient/families who are in the Hospice home care program
2. "Pre-terminal" patients not yet eligible for admission into the Hospice home care program, but in need of some Hospice support services. Includes patients who are (usually) aware of their diagnoses and still undergoing curative treatment such as chemotherapy, radiation, or hyperalimentation
3. The patient whose terminal condition has stabilized, and is not presently in the Hospice home care program but can benefit from supportive day care.

All admissions depend upon the resources of the Hospice program and an evaluation of the participant's appropriateness for day care (Seely 1990).

Transportation

Various means of transportation can be used, depending upon the location, finances, and resources of the individual Hospice providing the day care program.

- Family may be responsible for arrangements to bring patient to and from day care
- Hospice volunteers (or other qualified community volunteers)
- Community transportation systems (such as hospital or nursing home transports, senior citizen or community center vans)
- Public transportation
- Hospice-owned van
- Contracted van/ambulette.

Who Pays for Hospice Day Care?

1. Medicare acknowledges that Hospice day care is an acceptable type of extended care; however, it is *not* a mandated service. Certified Hospice programs receive the regular Medicare reimbursement at the usual "routine home care rate" when Hospice day care is specified in the patient's plan of care; however, there is *no* additional reimbursement for this day care service.

2. In addition, according to Henderson and Holden, some Hospices have been successful ". . . obtaining reimbursement for day care from commercial carriers and health maintenance organizations. . . " ("Hospice Day Care"). More education is needed, documenting the effectiveness and value of Hospice day care, to encourage more third-party payors to provide coverage for Hospice day care.

Those Hospice programs that charge day care participants charge on a sliding scale, according to ability to pay. Donations are needed to cover care of the indigent patient. Volunteer services and in-kind donations help purchase needed medical supplies and other equipment.

Advantages

- Offers opportunities for patients to get out of the house and be with other people
- Enhances quality of life for patients and families
- The patient/family have a choice of activities and days
- Program hours can be flexible to meet individual needs (from regular day hours to "after hours")
- Can be part of a caregiver support system, offering a safe, life-affirming environment for the patient
    - Provides respite for caregivers, such as the elderly, the physically limited, the stressed-out and sleep-deprived
    - Enables caregiver to continue to work and take care of chores and other responsibilities
    - Enables children/grandchildren to attend school, do homework, and participate in peer activities
    - Part-time caregiver can be used
- Provides an outlet for patients to use their talents and skills, to document and record life experiences and leave something behind for their families and significant others: creative arts (painting, sculpture, journal, music composition, poetry, drama, making audio and video tapes) (See also "What Are Some of the Things a Patient and Family Might Do to Maximize the Time That Is Left?" in Chapter 2.)
- Can be a center for Hospice services and provide counseling, intensive therapies, and treatments with equipment on site
- Often can eliminate need for a home care nurse and other therapist home visits
- An established Hospice day care program can provide services to the larger community within the resources of the individual program
- Extends the continuum of care and can become a routine Hospice service in the future
- Can provide for earlier Hospice admissions by getting referrals earlier.

While only a few Hospice programs provide such services at present, Hospice day care can be part of community outreach. "Continued education of the public and the medical community about the viability [cost effectiveness] and legitimacy of Hospice day care is greatly needed" (Henderson and Holden, 1991).

References

Henderson, Lee Ann, and Connie Holden, "Hospice Day Care," in *Alternative Care Programs in Hospice* (Arlington, VA: National Hospice Organization, Inc. [Alternative Care Task Force], 1991), pp. 13-15.

Seely, Sondra, "Why Hospice Day Care" *The American Journal of Hospice Care,* (January/February 1990), pp. 16-17.

Sendor, Virginia F., Observations (Unpublished): On-Site Hospice Visits (including Day Care Programs).

Webb, Trudy, Executive Director. Hospice by the Sea, Inc., Boca Raton, FL, 1991. (In this independent freestanding Hospice, located in a specially designed and constructed building, the day care area is adjacent to the inpatient unit.)

Wurth, Christopher, Administrator, St. Peter's Hospice, Albany, NY, 1990. (This hospital-based Hospice program has beds in a dedicated Hospice inpatient unit. The day care area is located adjacent to the Hospice area in the hospital.)

Q: What is meant by "drugs and biologicals" in a Medicare certified Hospice program?

Drugs and biologicals is the term used to cover all kinds of medications that exist at this time or in the future. In a Medicare certified Hospice program, drugs and biologicals are used for palliative/comfort care in the treatment of the terminal illness and related conditions involving pain control and symptom management.

All biologicals are drugs, but not all drugs are biologicals.

Drugs usually refer to medications that are chemically created in the pharmaceutical laboratory.

Biologicals are organic in nature and cultured in the laboratory from a living organism—bacteria and/or tissue culture (animal or plant)—with fractions of the product extracted for medicinal use. Examples are serums, vaccines, and immunosuppressing medications, including antibodies, antitoxins, antigens, etc., used in the prevention or treatment of the disease.

Frequently, there is an overlap between drugs and biologicals. Allergic reactions to some of the original organic biologicals, as well as the expense and perhaps some difficulty in obtaining and controlling limited supply sources, led to ongoing scientific research. As a result, some medications that formerly were strictly biologic in origin now can be "modified biologicals" and chemically replicated in the laboratory. (Examples are insulin, penicillin, and tetanus.)

When questions arise, check with the patient's physician or pharmacist, as well as appropriate Hospice staff.

Reference

Pardo, Benjamin, R.Ph., Barley's Pharmacy, Inc. (Westbury, NY: Private communication, 1992).

Q: What is the difference between a Hospice and a regular home health agency?

Regulations and licensing governing Hospices and home health agencies may vary from state to state.

Hospice care is very different from other home health care. Most home health agency services are utilized when a patient has physical limitations and/or skilled nursing or teaching needs after discharge from the hospital. There is emphasis on skilled nursing, rehabilitative, or restorative therapies. A home health agency's involvement tends to move from more frequent to less frequent visits. Hospice services actually increase with the patient's declining health and the subsequent rising family stress. Hospice offers interdisciplinary care with the added benefit of case management and continuity of care across multiple settings [in the home, or contracted care in a hospital, nursing home, or special residential facility]. Hospice care provides services to the patient and the family, including bereavement services. Hospice services provide pain and symptom control, and make the promise that patients do not have to die in pain or die alone.

Reference

Commercial Reimbursement Insurance Monograph (Arlington, VA: National Hospice Organization, Inc. [NHO Commercial Reimbursement Task Force], 1991).

Q: What is the difference between a Medicare Hospice program and a palliative care program?

In *both* the Medicare Hospice Program and the Palliative Care Program, the *type* of care provided is palliative. It is comfort care, provided when cure is no longer possible. What is *different* in the programs reflects the Medicare regulations, scope, and restraints imposed upon a Medicare certified Hospice program. Palliative care programs provide a broader interpretation of the Hospice philosophy and principles prior to and after the Medicare Hospice Benefit.

The main benefit of the licensed and certified Medicare Hospice is that terminally ill patients and their families receive comprehensive Hospice care from a provider who not only specializes in the care of the dying and the bereaved, but is also responsible for the total patient/family plan of care. The Hospice is responsible for the patient, whether the plan of care calls for the patient to be at home, in a hospital or nursing home, a day care center, or elsewhere, regardless of the site of services. This may or may not be so in a palliative care program.

A palliative care program may or may not be licensed, and may or may not offer *all* the services provided by the Hospice. While the same compassionate comfort care is provided in both programs, the *admission criteria differ*.

- To be admitted into the Medicare Hospice program, the prognosis must be six months or less to live. This prognosis must be certified by both the patient's primary physician and the Hospice medical director.
- The patients in the palliative care program may or may not be at the end-stage of their illness. While they usually are medically diagnosed as having a terminal illness, their condition may be chronic or may have become stabilized.
- In the palliative care program, the patient may be receiving active treatment such as chemotherapy and hope is for a remission, if not actual cure.
- In the Medicare Hospice program, the patient chooses to forego the standard Medicare benefits (for the terminal illness and related conditions) and opts for the Hospice Medicare Benefit instead. This benefit is provided only in a Hospice program certified by Medicare. *However, the stand-*

ard Medicare benefit also will help pay for covered costs necessary to treat an unrelated condition.

- In the Hospice program, it is implied that a primary care person or support system will be available to the patient. Some Hospice programs will not accept a patient who does not have a primary caregiver available. In a palliative care program, a primary care person is preferred but not required. (See also "Why Is Having a Primary Caregiver So Important to the Patient in a Hospice Program?" in Chapter 2.)

Medicare Hospice regulations state that at least 80 percent of their patients must be in the home care component of the Hospice program and no more than 20 percent can be in a hospital or nursing home. This is not applicable in a palliative care program.

Hospice bills under the Medicare/Medicaid Hospice Benefits. For those patients who are not eligible for Medicare or Medicaid, Hospices also can bill for Hospice benefits from commercial insurance companies and health maintenance organizations (HMOs). The palliative care program bills under traditional, regular health care reimbursement, depending upon the individual insurance coverage for each patient. Both programs do provide services to the medically indigent.

Despite these differences, there are similarities in both Hospice and palliative care programs. The common goal is to provide the palliative care that will enable the patient, the family, and significant others to be as comfortable as possible for whatever time is left.

Both programs are concerned with:

- Pain management and symptom control
- Relief from suffering
- Enhancing the quality of life
- The patient, the family, and significant others are considered to be the "unit of care" and are invited to give input to the individual patient's plan of care.

Both programs recognize that some patients and families may have difficulty in acknowledging that the patient is in the terminal stage. Respecting patient and family issues and following Hospice philosophy and principles of care assures competent medical treatment for the patient. Family structures may vary. In coming to the realization of the terminal condition of the patient, palliative care may assist in the later admission to a Hospice.

Denial is a coping behavior in some cases; patients know they are dying (although they may choose not to talk about it) and may insist on continuing aggressive treatment until the end. In these cases, neither Hospice nor palliative care may be acceptable to the patient and family (example: AIDS patients).

Palliative care follows the Hospice philosophy and principles but does not have the restraints of place of service and length of time dictated by prognosis. The patient may receive active but not aggressive treatment under the palliative care program.

Hospice and palliative care are not mutually exclusive of each other; it is the interpretation of the terms by various settings that may cause confusion. Whichever program is chosen, what is important is that the patient and family will receive appropriate and compassionate professional medical care during this crucial period of their lives.

10
VOLUNTEERS

1. What is the difference between Hospice staff and volunteers?
2. What do Hospice volunteers do?
3. What does the volunteer Hospice governing board of directors/trustees do?
4. What are some examples of the professionals who volunteer in the Hospice program?
5. How qualified are these volunteers—and others—to work for Hospice? What about those volunteers who will come into my home? Who provides their training?
6. Does volunteer training stop after their graduation? Who supervises these volunteers?
7. What exactly do these "good neighbor" volunteers do when they come into my home?
8. What are some examples of "good neighbor" volunteer placement?
9. What do bereavement volunteers do? Can any volunteer become a bereavement volunteer?
10. Are there some things volunteers are not permitted to do?
11. What about confidentiality?
12. I would like to see an example of a "Volunteer Interest Form."
13. I might be interested—what does a "Hospice Volunteer Application" look like?

Q: What is the difference between Hospice staff and volunteers?

Paid Hospice employees are qualified staff who are financially compensated for providing their professional expertise to the Hospice program. They must meet all professional requirements in their particular discipline.

Hospice volunteers are also considered staff; however, they are not paid for the particular expertise they share, whether in the office, or as a "Good Neighbor" volunteer in the patient's home, or in any other capacity. They also must provide all professional certification when indicated, must meet the same health requirements as paid staff, and are covered by the same insurance provided by many Hospice programs.

The patient/family ("Good Neighbor") volunteer is an integral part of the Hospice health care team and is expected to participate in the design of the plan of care, to participate at team meetings, case updates, and ongoing supervision contacts with the coordinator of volunteers.

According to the National Hospice Organization "Fact Sheet" (1995), ". . . Hospices employ more than 25,000 paid professionals. . . . 96,000 volunteers—75,000 female, 21,000 male—contributed approximately 5.25 million hours of service in 1992 . . . [and] 55 percent of Hospice patient/families accept volunteer services."

Reference

National Hospice Organization, "Hospice Fact Sheet" (Arlington, VA: Updated October 10, 1995).

Q: What do Hospice volunteers do?

Because reimbursement levels for Hospice services are inadequate, volunteers provide invaluable assistance in many areas of the Hospice program. Reimbursement by both government and third-party payors does not cover the costs of providing the services mandated by the Hospice philosophy and required by federal law for all Medicare/Medicaid certified programs. Federal law mandates that Hospice volunteers provide at least 5 percent of all staff hours worked, regardless of the tax status of the Hospice.

Historically, in some smaller Hospice programs, volunteers provided more than 50 percent of the services provided. Indeed, some were all-volunteer programs, particularly during the early "start-up" phase.

Today, in the larger Medicare/Medicaid certified programs, volunteers regularly provide about 15 percent of all hours worked for Hospice.

By donating their caring and expertise, volunteers help ensure the smooth functioning of the Hospice program, both in the administrative area and in helping directly with the patients, families, and significant others. By participating directly in the program, volunteers enhance community outreach, encouraging community awareness and participation in the work of Hospice.

Considered by many to be "the heart of Hospice," volunteers serve in five major categories:

1. office assistance
2. as "Good Neighbor" volunteers (with direct patient/family contact)
3. as bereavement volunteers
4. as professionals providing their expertise without pay
5. as members of the Hospice governing Board of Directors/Trustees.

Fifty-nine percent of volunteer hours are provided in direct support of patients (through direct patient/family care or through bereavement services); 41 percent of volunteer hours are spent in administrative support.

. . . [Usually required to make a one-year commitment, the] average volunteer provides volunteer services for three years. Fifty percent of Hospice volunteers stay for six or more years.

. . . Volunteers are recruited from many sources: churches [and synagogues]; civic groups; social groups; professional organizations; business and industry; and colleges and secondary schools ("Fact Sheet," 1995).

In addition to saving the Hospice needed dollars on a tight budget, the "Good Neighbor" patient/family volunteer can play a critical role (*Policies and Procedures for Volunteers*, 1988). For example, the volunteer frequently has more contact with the patient and family than do other members of the Hospice team. The volunteer immediately reports any change in the patient's condition—to the coordinator of volunteers or the patient's Hospice nurse—if the patient is not eating or sleeping, is having pain, or seems in any way changed or uncomfortable from the volunteer's previous visit. These reports may be crucial in assuring the patient's physical and psychological comfort and the family's ability to cope with the impact of the illness.

References

National Hospice Organization, "Hospice Fact Sheet" (Arlington, VA: Updated October 10, 1995).

Policies and Procedures for Volunteers (Hempstead, NY: Long Island Foundation for Hospice Care and Research, Inc., 1988).

Q: What does the volunteer Hospice governing board of directors/trustees do?

The volunteer board of directors/trustees of the Hospice organization manages the affairs and controls the finances, including the investment of its funds, establishes the policies of the agency, and supervises the continuity of its services (*By-laws*, 1988). It is the responsibility of the board to take all necessary steps to carry out the purposes of the agency according to the law (federal, state, and local) and as provided in the certificate of incorporation and the operating certificate granted by the state department of health. The board adopts and authorizes an annual operating budget; determines, approves, implements, and monitors all policies and procedures for patient/family care; approves all contracts with the agency; and ensures that all services provided are consistent with accepted standards of practice.

The board also employs an executive director who is responsible to the board for the current and future programs of the Hospice and its day-to-day management.

References

By-laws, (Hempstead, NY: Long Island Foundation for Hospice Care and Research, Inc., 1988).

Federal Conditions of Participation (42 C.F.R. Part 418.5) for Medicare Certified Programs, Washington, DC.

Q: What are some examples of the professionals who volunteer in the Hospice program?

Recognizing the needs of an individual Hospice program, some volunteers may be professionals who choose to provide their expertise without pay. For example, a skilled licensed nurse may volunteer to be an on-call or backup nurse. A social worker specializing in bereavement may donate services as a consultant to the Hospice staff, help in the interviewing process for staff acquisition, or provide bereavement support and in-service training sessions for staff and volunteers. A physician—medical doctor or osteopathic physician—may volunteer his or her services when the medical director or Hospice physician is on vacation or heavily involved in a peak caseload. Or an attorney may provide legal expertise *pro bono*, working with contracts, leasing agreements, or other legal matters. A corporate vice president of human resources or a director of personnel may donate expertise in updating the Hospice personnel policies and procedures. An accountant may guide a Hospice program through the process and provide the paperwork in acquiring the Internal Revenue Service 501(c)(3) tax-exempt status. Or the owner of a private employment agency may volunteer professional expertise for the required credential checking for candidates seeking employment in the Hospice program. An artist may donate design and layouts for brochures, and a printer may donate the paper, printing and folding.

There are many caring members of the larger community who help various Hospice programs in different ways.

Q: How qualified are these volunteers—and others— to work for Hospice? What about those volunteers who will come into my home? Who provides their training?

Hospice programs provide special training for all their volunteers in all categories.

Volunteers must meet the same health requirements as the paid staff. They must have the same pre-employment health examination form completed, dated, and signed by the examining physician. And they must submit a background resume and at least three references. Each is checked, documented, and placed in the volunteer's personnel file. Also checked and documented are any professional licenses or other credentials (if applicable), including current driver's license and insurance coverage for the car they drive on Hospice business.

The length of the Hospice volunteer training program may vary from fifteen to thirty-six hours, depending on the individual Hospice, its size, and the extent of the services provided.

In addition to an introduction and orientation into the individual Hospice program, volunteers are required to attend training seminars led by medical and mental health experts, social workers, clergy, and other specialists who provide insights on how to address the physical, social, emotional, spiritual, and other practical support needs of the patients, their families, and significant others. Similar training sessions are conducted for members of the Hospice governing boards of directors/trustees.

A graduation usually is part of the last session of this initial training program. In a "Celebration of Life," these new volunteers are welcomed into the expanding Hospice program by others participating in the festivities: perhaps some members of the Hospice staff, the governing board, and existing volunteers. Some Hospices also encourage the volunteers to invite a member of their family to attend the festivities.

Individual post-training interviews are conducted, usually by the coordinator of volunteers. If the volunteer has met all the requirements, an active volunteer assignment will be made, either in the office or as a "Good Neighbor" volunteer in the field. A match is made between the needs of the patient/family, the Hospice needs, and the interests of the volunteer.

Volunteers usually are asked to make a time commitment to the Hospice program for at least one year after completing the training program, to donate approximately four hours a week, to attend the monthly mutual support meetings, and ongoing periodic inservice training sessions. Volunteers are also asked to attend appropriate team meetings.

Q: Does volunteer training stop after their graduation? Who supervises these volunteers?

No, volunteer training does not stop after graduation. The needs of patients and families are not static; they change with the ebb and flow of the terminal illness. Volunteers may experience various reactions and perhaps some feelings of inadequacy. Therefore, volunteer attendance is mandated at monthly mutual support meetings. Participants are encouraged to share their experiences and concerns with each other, with the coordinator of volunteers, and with other appropriate Hospice staff. These support groups for volunteers include supervision, education, case reporting, and planning.

Most programs also provide periodic ongoing inservice training, which includes issues of concern such as updates on the care of AIDS patients, substance abuse, and working with dysfunctional families. Office volunteers are encouraged to attend these sessions, too.

Special education and training sessions are provided for the governing board of directors/trustees.

Volunteers must continue to abide by all health regulations. They must document their volunteer activity in accordance with established Hospice procedures. Volunteer logs and other forms are provided and reviewed by the coordinator of volunteers.

Volunteer performance is usually reviewed formally within three months after beginning work as a volunteer, again after six months, and once a year thereafter. Involved in this review will be the coordinator of volunteers, the volunteer, and appropriate staff.

What do office volunteers do?

One office volunteer had worked for an actuary before retirement. She shared her actuarial skills to design record-keeping reports and summaries. Her charts and tables were used for presentations, including patient/family profiles and volunteer program updates. She also kept the attendance records and tracked overtime, compensatory time, and vacation time.

A retired executive secretary shared her skills, helping the hospice executive director prepare special grants and other documents. Her dictation, transcription, typing, and organizational skills were of great help. She also was able to work independently in doing some telephone follow-up.

The office support volunteer application (see Appendix A, Figure 15) indicates some of the areas in which office assistance may be needed.

Q: What exactly do these "good neighbor" volunteers do when they come into my home?

"Good Neighbor" volunteer services are various emotional and practical assistance measures that volunteers are trained to provide to assist a terminal patient and the patient's family members/significant others. These volunteers are trained in a special Hospice volunteer-training program and perform chores and provide support to patient/families short of skilled health care and professional counseling. Examples of volunteer services are:

Compassionate listening helps patient and family members express their feelings, communicate openly together, process issues related to death and dying, and feel supported in the struggle and transition they are going through. Compassionate listening and support continues through the bereavement phase. *Note:* Since living with dignity in the midst of serious illness, dying itself, and bereavement are all essentially natural processes, normal and natural friendship, openness, and listening are critically important support services to dying patients and their families. For this reason, a volunteer component is a federal requirement for all Medicare certified Hospice programs.

Respite Care involves the volunteer staying with the patient while the family caregiver leaves the home for a period of time. This service enables caregivers to obtain relief from the emotionally and physically draining responsibility of 24-hour care for the patient.

Transportation is provided to escort and deliver the patient and/or family members to appointments, recreation activities that otherwise would be impossible, and special events that provide quality of life to the patient and family. Transportation also includes picking up groceries and any other items to help the family manage.

Internal and external chores are done to help the patient and family in the home and the general community. Chores might be housecleaning, custodial care of the patient, delivering items, arranging for church/synagogue involvement, or any other practical matter.

24-hour reassurance is provided by volunteers. The patient and family know that the "Good Neighbor" Hospice volunteer is always available. Many times, more than one volunteer is assigned to a patient/family to ensure that support is available any time of day or night. Sometimes the volunteer is present at the actual time of death.

References

DiSorbo, Philip G., Exec. Dir., Capital District Hospice (Schenectady, NY: Private communications, 1989).

Policies and Procedures for Volunteers and *Volunteer Manual* (Hempstead, NY: Long Island Foundation for Hospice Care and Research, Inc., 1988).

Q: What are some examples of "good-neighbor" volunteer placement? (Adjusted to protect confidentiality.)

Volunteer Placement Number 1

A mother had died and the funeral had just been held. The 34-year-old widower was coping with three children ages four, six, and eight. The volunteer was a tenured fifth-grade schoolteacher. Her original assignment was to visit the family after school twice a week to help the children with their homework and get them ready for bed.

This gave the distraught father a bit of time for himself to take care of some of his own needs without taking time off from his job. He could visit the dentist or do a bit of personal shopping, spend a bit of time with family or friends, or just go upstairs to his room for some needed respite and quiet time after a hectic day at work, secure in the knowledge that his children were being supervised, their homework completed satisfactorily, and they had their baths and their "story hour." Rested and energized, the father could then help put his children to bed.

A second volunteer was assigned to this family, so the teacher-volunteer could attend open school night with the father and go to additional meetings with the children's teachers and the school psychologist, to help eliminate some behavioral and academic problems stemming from the mother's lingering death from cancer over a two-year period. Together, these two volunteers visited the family four afternoons and/or evenings a week. One volunteer looked after the children while the other provided academic help. During this traumatic time, the father and his three children were able to spend some special time together. About eighteen months later, the widower remarried and his children had a new "mother."

Volunteer Placement Number 2

The wife had died in the hospital. The course of her cancer required chemotherapy, radiation, stays in the hospital, and some time at home with brief periods of remission. With both daughters grown, living elsewhere, and working full-time, the widower felt bereft and very much alone. As a retired businessman, he had financial resources and was accustomed to handling his own business matters; however, he could not cope with handling all the medical bills and household expenses. He could not sleep and "retreated" from his adult children.

Hospice was called in during the wife's last week in the hospital. A male volunteer, also a retired businessman, was assigned, with the days and hours to be agreed upon. After several visits, a rapport was established. The men would go for walks together or to the local diner to eat, "Dutch treat." The volunteer met both daughters and together they began to organize the financial papers and address other pertinent matters. Gradually, the widower joined them. Some incorrect bills were corrected and paid. The insurance company was notified and documentation mailed. Records and files were organized and the family attorney and accountant were contacted. Phone calls were made, appointments set up. Follow-up correspondence and calls also were made to expedite the process. Eventually, all was straightened out and the two men went fishing again and again. They continued to stay in touch with occasional lunches and have invited their daughters to join them for dinner for special "memory" events and "anniversaries."

Volunteer Placement Number 3

Both parents had AIDS and were intravenous drug abusers. Their six-year-old daughter was not HIV positive. The father had just died of AIDS; the mother was participating in the local methadone program and was in and out of the hospital. The grandparents lived at a distance and felt they could not help.

The assigned volunteer was a mother whose son had died of AIDS a few years ago. Her original assignment was to baby-sit the child for four hours at a time, while the mother attended sessions at the methadone clinic twice a week. Circumstances led the volunteer to be with the child for eight to ten hours a day, four days a week, instead of as originally scheduled and agreed upon in the plan of care with the Hospice coordinator of volunteers, the volunteer, and the child's mother. Instead of just spending time in the playground and then going back to the apartment, the volunteer planned some special activities for the child. They had picnics at the park, took trips to the zoo, and went to the movies to see a Walt Disney film.

At one point, the mother did not return at all after she left home to visit the methadone clinic. The volunteer took the child into her own home for two days until Hospice staff were able to locate the mother, who had *not* gone to the methadone clinic. The mother had become confused, felt ill, and checked herself into the AIDS clinic at the local hospital, where she died three days later. The volunteer continued to take care of the child while Hospice staff located the grandparents and helped make the necessary funeral and other arrangements. Sessions were set up with both the maternal and paternal grandparents to help them work through their feelings of anguish and grief. The maternal grandparents agreed to take care of the child. Since they lived in another state, Hospice turned the case over to the department of social services in that area. The volunteer has kept in touch with occasional phone calls to the child, greeting cards, and little gifts at holiday time.

Q: What do bereavement volunteers do? Can any volunteer become a bereavement volunteer?

Bereavement volunteers provide emotional support to bereaved family members through the bereavement stage. (See "What Is 'Bereavement'?" and "What Are Some of the Grief Reactions the Family May Experience When Someone Dies?" in Chapter 11.)

Frequently, a close personal relationship develops between the "Good Neighbor" volunteer and the family, and continues after the patient's death. The volunteer is assigned a schedule of contacts with the family. This may include attending the wake and the funeral—alone or with other Hospice team members—as well as post-funeral condolence calls and continued contact with the family for up to thirteen months after the patient's death.

Visits, telephone calls, and the exchange of cards and letters provide emotional support to the family during their bereavement. This continued contact with bereaved family members is an important element of the Hospice philosophy—to help family members through the transition period as they work through their loss. It also helps the volunteer deal with his or her own sense of grief.

A volunteer who has been active in the Hospice program for at least six months usually has learned to develop compassionate listening skills. This volunteer—who is sensitive to the needs of patient/family and significant others, who accepts them just as they are, who can be completely nonjudgmental and "be there" for the family—can be a successful bereavement volunteer.

Q: Are there some things volunteers are not permitted to do?

Volunteers may *not* provide any hands-on care to patients; they may *not* administer medication to patients. On-duty volunteers may *not* be under the influence of alcohol or involved in substance abuse. Volunteers may *not* speak to the media without clearing it first with the coordinator of volunteers and receiving written permission in advance.

Occasionally, individuals or groups express appreciation for services provided with an offer of a gift to the volunteer(s). A volunteer may *not* accept a gift in excess of $10 in value. It is appropriate to point out that a gift or donation to Hospice would be acceptable, perhaps a memorial gift or one in honor of a special occasion, or to help support a program of Hospice that was of great help to the patient/family.

Volunteers are asked *not* to smoke while in the home of a patient/family, even if others are smoking.

Before leaving the patient's home, the volunteer must always check to be sure that the patient is *not* left alone. If the patient is alone, the volunteer must notify the coordinator of volunteers or the primary nurse on call, who will advise the volunteer what to do.

If a conflict or lack of compatibility arises between the volunteers and the patient/family, this must be reported immediately to the coordinator of volunteers, who will evaluate the situation. It may be determined that it is *not* appropriate for this volunteer to remain on the case, and another volunteer will be assigned.

Reference

Policies and Procedures for Volunteers and *Volunteer Manual* (Hempstead, NY: Long Island Foundation for Hospice Care and Research, Inc., 1988).

Q: What about confidentiality?

Strict confidentiality is observed at all times. The Hospice program includes required interdisciplinary team meetings, mutual support sessions, and ongoing inservices. The goal is to provide the very best of compassionate care; to do whatever can be done to enhance the quality of life for the patients, families, and significant others. These discussions frequently lead directly to changes in the patient/family plan of care.

All staff—whether paid or volunteer, full-time or part-time, administrative or directly involved in patient and family care—must adhere to the strict Hospice policy of confidentiality and must sign a memorandum of understanding regarding this policy, which is in force at all times. Any violation of this confidentiality is grounds for immediate dismissal from the Hospice program.

Examples of the memoranda for Hospice staff and volunteers follow:

Memorandum of Understanding for Hospice Personnel

I understand that any information concerning patient/family care, treatment, condition or personal data is considered absolutely confidential and may not be discussed with anyone other than those directly responsible for Hospice care and treatment including authorized consultants and/or contractors, and volunteers who are directly involved in the care of the patient/family. This includes, but is not limited to, information about patients' names, diagnoses, treatment of special family problems.

Name: _____
      (Signature)   (Please print)   (Date)

Memorandum of Understanding for Hospice Volunteers

I understand that I will be exposed to information of a confidential nature pertaining to patient/families in the course of my volunteer work with Hospice. I further understand that this information is strictly confidential and that I will discuss it only with Hospice staff and volunteers who are directly involved in the care of the patient/family. This includes, but is not limited to, information about patients' names, addresses, diagnoses, treatment of special family problems.

Name: _____
     (Signature)   (Please print)   (Date)

References

Hospice Operations Manual (Hempstead, NY: Long Island Foundation for Hospice Care and Research, Inc., 1988).

Volunteer Manual (Hempstead, NY: Long Island Foundation for Hospice Care and Research, Inc., 1988), 199-201.

Q: I would like to see an example of a "Volunteer Interest Form."

A sample form is shown in Appendix A as Figure 16. Other elements can be added to the form to tailor it to the needs of the Hospice and/or its patients.

Q: What does a "Hospice Volunteer Application" look like?

A sample application for a Hospice volunteer is shown in Appendix A as Figure 17.

11
BEREAVEMENT

1. What is bereavement?
2. What are some of the grief reactions the family may experience when someone dies?
3. What are some of the factors that determine grief responses?
4. What is meant by mourning? When is it finished?
5. Isn't it morbid to talk about funeral arrangements before the death?
6. What are some of the reactions that one may expect from children when there is a death in the family?
7. What is the role of children during the funeral?
8. What do you tell children about death?
9. How can children become involved when the patient is in the Hospice program?
10. What is meant by "anticipatory grief"?
11. How does the Hospice offer bereavement services?

Q: What is bereavement?

Webster defines *bereavement* as a "loss of a loved one by death" (*Webster's Unabridged Dictionary,* 1966). Bereavement is a complex issue, and people experience their grief in many varied ways. Webster also defines *grief* as "an intense emotional suffering caused by loss."

Since the patient, family, and significant others are considered the "unit of care," Hospice programs are committed to providing bereavement services to the family after the patient's death. To implement these support services, the Hospice interdisciplinary team addresses the issues of each family member and significant others with an individual plan of care. Development of the plan is based on the needs as expressed by the patient and family during the "anticipatory grief" stage, and by the family and significant others during the period following the death of the patient. (See also "What is meant by 'Anticipatory Grief'?" in this chapter.)

Reference

Webster's Unabridged Dictionary (Springfield, Mass.: Merriam-Webster Inc., 1966), pp. 206, 999.

Q: What are some of the grief reactions the family may experience when someone dies?

> You cannot prevent the birds of sorrow
> From flying over your head.
> But you can prevent them
> From building nests in your hair.
> —Chinese proverb

Initially you may feel intense shock, disbelief, and a sense of numbness.

Don't be surprised by symptoms such as:

- Headaches
- Extreme fatigue
- Loss of appetite
- Weight loss
- Feelings of a lump in the throat
- Shortness of breath
- Sleeplessness or restlessness
- Limited attention span
- Forgetfulness
- Changes in concentration
- Memory loss or confusion
- Inability to organize your day.

Feelings such as anger, guilt, or resentment are normal.

The grieving process can be an intensely disorganizing experience, so much so that some people say they feel they're "going crazy" or think they see or hear the deceased.

Sometimes people dream about their deceased loved one being alive or smell his or her cologne. These experiences are all quite normal, should they occur.

Sudden or unexpected events may trigger a renewed sense of sadness and grief. Allow this to run its course.

Crying is a necessary and healthy way to express grief. Don't be ashamed or afraid to cry often and share your feelings with others. This is highly therapeutic.

You may find yourself reminiscing about your loved one often—this can be very healing. Allow friends, family, and others to help and support you. Seek the help and company of others: family, friends, clergy, health professionals, or grief support groups.

You will also need time to be alone to sort through thoughts, memories, and emotions.

The use of alcohol and drugs will only numb your sense of loss temporarily and may prolong your grief.

A physical check-up during the first few months is a good idea, especially if any physical symptoms persist.

Grieving requires energy and time. Grieving associated with sudden death may require *more* energy and time.

Give yourself time to adjust. If possible, avoid major changes in your life.

Grieving is a process that may continue for many months and can ultimately result in personal growth.

Grieving is an intensely personal experience. You may or may not have any of the symptoms listed. *Your* situation is unique; *your* response is unique.

You may feel you have "gotten over" your grief, only to see it recur. This is normal.

Reference

Palliative Care Manual (New York: St. Luke's/Roosevelt Hospital Center, 1990).

Q: What are some of the factors that determine grief responses?

There are many different ways that death can affect family dynamics and each individual member. For some, grief is an intense experience; for others, it may be rather mild. Grieving may begin when the reality of the prognosis is perceived, or some may not experience grief until sometime after the death. The time-frame for grief may be short or may involve a prolonged period of time. There is no "normal" length of time for the grieving process; it is completely individual.

Some of the factors that the Hospice interdisciplinary team considers when assessing family members for bereavement support are: What was the relationship of the deceased to each member? What was the nature of the attachment? Was it positive or negative? Was it strong? Were security issues involved? Was there ambivalence in the relationship? When and where the patient died may also influence the grief reaction. What has been the family's history of loss, and how did they handle losses in the past?

Reactions of family members vary and depend upon their changing role in the family dynamics, as well as age, sex, and coping skills. Social, religious/spiritual, and maturity factors also affect how each person grieves.

Q: What is meant by mourning? When is it finished?

After the death of a family member, the tasks of mourning must be accomplished for grief to be complete. J. W. Worden outlines the four tasks of mourning:

(1) To accept the reality of the loss: the person is gone and will not return.
(2) To experience the pain of grief: not everyone experiences the same intensity of pain or feels it in the same way, but it is impossible to lose someone you have been attached to without expressing some level of pain.
(3) To adjust to an environment in which the deceased is missing: this will mean different things to each person depending on the role of the deceased.
(4) To withdraw emotional energy and reinvest it in another relationship: the fourth task is hindered by holding on to the past attachment rather than going on and forming new ones. For many people, task 4 is the most difficult one to accomplish.

One of the landmarks of completed grief reaction is when the person is able to think of the deceased without pain.

There is no set time for these tasks to be completed, but some feel that it takes a full year before grief begins to abate.

Reference

Worden, J. W., *Grief Counseling and Grief Therapy* (New York: Springer, 1982).

Q: Isn't it morbid to talk about funeral arrangements before the death?

No. It is rather a gesture of love and respect to make such arrangements when they can be done "care-fully." When you write a will or purchase life insurance, you are making preparation for the financial security of those you love; and, similarly, making funeral arrangements is making preparation for emotional confidence and spiritual satisfaction. Ask yourself the question whether this should be done in haste at the time of death when everyone is emotionally distressed, or beforehand when you can weigh the options and discuss them with all concerned (Dransfield, 1991).

A major part of the role of Hospice is to assist the patient, family, and significant others in dealing with the issues addressed in the total plan of care. These discussions may include what to do about funeral arrangements and will reflect and respect the culture and lifestyles of the patient and families, including differences between them, if any.

Reference

Dransfield, Rev. S. L., "Sooner Is Better." Unpublished. (Hempstead, NY: Long Island Foundation for Hospice Care and Research, Inc., 1991).

Q: What are some of the reactions that one may expect from children when there is a death in the family?

Each child will react in a different manner. Reactions will depend on the age of the child, psychosocial development, relationship with the dead person, and the child's history of loss. The child's reaction also depends upon how prepared the child has been during the terminal illness, as well as the reaction of the family to the death.

Dan Schaefer outlines some of the behavior that may occur: exhaustion, dependency, feelings of unreality, panic, preoccupation with the dead person, hyperactivity, destructive behavior, and regression.

Dr. John Bowlby, who has worked with bereaved children, observed that there are three stages of grief that most children go through: protest, pain, and hope.

> It's important to remember that all of the feelings associated with grief ebb and flow, and that the child will inevitably go back over these emotions time and again. We love to neatly compartmentalize things, to finish with one, then go on to the next. But it doesn't work that way with the emotions of grief (Schaefer and Lyons, 1986).

References

Bowlby, J., *Attachments, Separation, and Loss* (New York: Basic Books, 1981).

Schaefer, D., and C. Lyons, *How Do We Tell The Children?* (New York: Newmarket Press, 1986).

Q: What is the role of children during the funeral?

Children should be involved in the planning of the funeral. The level of involvement of each child should be decided by the child, not by the adults in the family.

Children need guidelines, an explanation as to what is going to happen and how the family members will react, and advice on what is expected of them. This will make children more comfortable in this traumatic situation.

The Hospice staff and funeral director can provide suggestions as to special gestures that the child may want to include in the funeral. The family may ask the funeral director to arrange a "family time" at the funeral home so the children may share a private time of grieving and mutual comforting.

The child will need a compassionate listener who will "listen" with the heart to what the child is saying—as well as to all the nonverbal expressions—and be completely nonjudgmental and caring.

Q: What do you tell children about death?

Tell children the truth about what is happening to the patient during the illness. This will help prepare children for their loved one's death. There are many factors to be considered when dealing with children and death. The age and psychosocial development of the child will determine just how much the child can understand. What was the child's relationship to the patient? What kind of person is the child? How does the child respond to stress?

Euphemisms such as "God took him," "He went on a long trip," or "He went to sleep" are *not* helpful and might confuse the child and lead to all sorts of strange thoughts about death. Answer each question openly and honestly.

The role of Hospice is to assist the family in dealing with these issues. This is reflected in the plan of care.

Q: How can children become involved when the patient is in the Hospice program?

When the patient is in the Hospice program, the family is the "unit of care," and this includes children.

Children's involvement depends on several factors: age, relationship with the patient, history of losses, level of development of the child, and the total reaction of the family to the illness and the impending death.

Since each child is different, it is helpful to talk with each child individually. This allows the child to express what he or she is feeling without conflict with siblings. This assures the child that someone in the family knows just how he or she is feeling, and this person can be a resource to the child in the future when questions arise or when the child needs to express further concerns.

The Hospice assists the family in dealing with these matters and giving appropriate support, helping to open communication with the entire family, including the children.

Q: What is meant by "Anticipatory Grief"?

Anticipatory grief is grief that begins before the patient has died. It is a normal part of the grief experienced by both Hospice patients and families, since the patients may have a prolonged illness. Families may feel that thinking about the patient's death is wishing the patient dead. If the patient has been ill for a long time, the family may have mentally "buried the patient" or may be angry that the dying process is taking so long. Hospice staff can help the family acknowledge these feelings and deal with them. Hospice staff can help them to be nonjudgmental and not feel guilty about having these negative feelings, in order to continue open communication with the patient and among family members.

Dying patients also may experience anticipatory grief, although they may feel it in different ways.

"The family is losing one loved one. The patient who is dying often has many attachments in his own life and to that extent, will be losing many significant others all at one time" (Worden, 1982).

The role of Hospice is also to assist the patients in understanding what is happening to them and assist all involved in the anticipatory grief process: the patient, the family, and significant others.

Reference

Worden, J. W., *Grief Counseling and Grief Therapy* (New York: Springer, 1982).

Q: How does the Hospice offer bereavement services?

The Hospice begins bereavement services before the patient dies. Hospice staff and volunteers provide ongoing support to patients and family members, including support on issues relating to anticipatory grief. (See "What Is Meant by 'Anticipatory Grief'?" in this chapter.) Hospice staff discusses practical preparations for the death (wake, funeral, etc.) at an appropriate time during this period.

At the time of death, the Hospice team is available to the patient and family by a 24-hour on-call system. The on-call system is used to notify the appropriate staff if the death occurs during off hours. Whenever possible, a Hospice representative attends the wake and/or funeral. A note of condolence, along with appropriate bereavement literature, is usually mailed to the family within a short time after the patient's death.

The Hospice team reviews each patient's case following his or her death. This review includes an assessment of any special bereavement problems and the designation of staff members or volunteers to follow the family in bereavement.

Following the patient's death, periodic contact with family members is maintained through phone calls and/or home visits, based on the needs and desires of the family. Within the first three months of bereavement, an assessment is made pertaining to individual family needs. Support groups are offered periodically. Referrals, as appropriate, are made to widowed persons, such as: outside groups, Compassionate Friends, or other community support programs.

Memorial services are offered periodically for the bereaved. These services are also attended by Hospice staff and volunteers.

Usually thirteen (13) months after the death of the patient the family will be considered for closure from the bereavement service if they appear to have adjusted to the patient's death. The family can request further bereavement support after this period.

12
RESOURCES

1. How can I locate a Hospice program in my area?
2. Is there a state Hospice organization in my state?
3. Are there any other agencies that might be able to help me?
4. Can you suggest some books for me to read?

Q: How can I locate a Hospice program in my area?

The National Hospice Organization (NHO) estimates that in the United States, there are more than 2,500 Hospice programs offering Hospice care in all fifty states and Puerto Rico. It is estimated that Hospice programs served more than 340,000 terminally ill persons and their families in 1994 (October 1995).

To find out if there is a Hospice program in your area, you may contact:

1. Your physician
2. The nearest hospital (ask for the discharge planner or the social worker)
3. Your area health department and department of social services
4. Your state Hospice organization
5. Members of the clergy
6. A home health agency
7. The Visiting Nurses' Association

Information about home health services in your area is also available from the Cancer Information Service, 1-(800) 4-CANCER.

You can write or call special resource groups, agencies, and certain publications that can provide you with pertinent information. It will be helpful to have specific information available when you contact any of these groups, by mail or telephone. For the kind of information that will help the Hospice or agency staff to be of help to the individual patient, the family, and significant others, see sample forms in Appendix A: Figure 18 ("Telephone Inquiries for Hospice Services") and Figure 19 ("Hospice Intake Sheet").

References

National Hospice Organization, Inc. (NHO)
1901 North Moore Street, Suite 901
Arlington, VA 22209
(703) 243-5900
Hospice Helpline: 1-(800) 658-8898

National Hospice Organization, "Hospice Fact Sheet" (Arlington, VA: Updated October 10, 1995).

Q: Is there a state Hospice organization in my state?

Each of the fifty states has its own state Hospice organization. The following list was compiled by The National Hospice Organization for 1995-6. (The NHO updates its listing annually.)

For further information (including Hospice day care and residential facilities), and Hospice referrals for your area, call the NHO Hospice Helpline at 1-(800) 658-8898.

Reference

National Hospice Organization, Inc. (NHO), *The 1995-96 Guide to the Nation's Hospices*, 1901 North Moore Street, Suite 901, Arlington, VA 22209.

State Hospice Organizations

ALABAMA
Alabama Hospice Organization

Susan Smith
Executive Director
459 N Dean Rd
Auburn, AL 36830
(334) 826-1944
FAX (334) 826-1973

ALASKA
Hospice of Alaska

    Paula Sanders McCarron
    President
    c/o Hospice of Anchorage
    3605 Arctic Blvd., #555
    Anchorage, AK 99503
    (907) 561-5322
    FAX (907) 561-0334

ARIZONA
Arizona Hospice Organization

    Marilyn H. Pate
    President
    c/o Northland Hospice
    Box 997
    Flagstaff, AZ 86002-0997
    (520) 779-1227
    FAX (520) 779-5884

ARKANSAS
Arkansas State Hospice Assoc.

    James D. McDonald
    President
    c/o Washington Regional Medical Ctr HH & Hosp
    4209 Frontage Rd
    Fayetteville, AR 72703-1994
    1-(800) 400-2340
    FAX (501) 442-0991

CALIFORNIA
California State Hospice Assoc.

    Margaret Clausen
    Executive Director
    PO Box 160087
    2023 N St, Suite 205
    Sacramento, CA 95816

(916) 441-3770
FAX (916) 441-4720

COLORADO
Colorado State Hospice Org.

Brian C Hoag
President
c/o Hospice of Larimer County
5205 S College Ave
Fort Collins, CO 80525
(970) 226-6533
FAX (970) 226-6999

CONNECTICUT
Hospice Council of Connecticut

Judith Bigler
President
c/o VNA Hospice
103 Woodland St
Hartford, CT 06105-2457
(203) 525-7001
FAX (203) 278-0581

DELAWARE
Delaware Hospice, Inc.

Susan D Lloyd
Executive Director
c/o Delaware Hospice—Dover Office
Clayton Bldg
3515 Silverside Rd, Suite 100
Wilmington, DE 19810
(302) 478-5707
FAX (302) 479-2586

DISTRICT OF COLUMBIA
Hospice Council of Metro Washington

David English
President

c/o Hospice of Northern Virginia
6400 Arlington Blvd, Suite 1000
Falls Church, VA 22042
(703) 534-7070
FAX (703) 538-2163

FLORIDA
Florida Hospices, Inc.

Patrice C Moore
President
c/o Hospice of N Central Florida
3615 SW 13th St
PO Box 15235
Gainesville, FL 32604
(904) 378-2121
FAX (904) 378-4111

GEORGIA
Georgia Hopice Organization

M Sharon Smith
President
c/o Kennestone Regional Hospice
PO Box 1208
Marietta, GA 30061-9975
(404) 426-3131
FAX (404) 793-7925

HAWAII
Hawaii State Hospice Network
Steven A Kula
President
c/o Hospice Hawaii
445 Seaside, Suite 604
Honolulu, HI 96815-2676
(808) 924-9255
FAX (808) 922-9161

IDAHO
Idaho Hospice Organization

Victoria Mayer
President
c/o Family Hospice of Saint Joseph Reg Med Ctr
608 5th Avenue
Lewiston, ID 83501-0816
(208) 799-5275
FAX (208) 799-5343

ILLINOIS
Illinois State Hospice Org.

Rosemary Crowley
Executive Director
1525 East 53rd St, Suite 720
Chicago, IL 60615
(312) 324-8844
FAX (312) 324-8247

INDIANA
Indiana Association of Hospices

Sharon O'Morrow
Executive Director
2142 W 86th Street
Indianapolis, IN 46260-1902
(317) 338-4716
FAX (317) 338-4038

IOWA
Iowa Hospice Organization

Linda Todd
President
c/o Hospice of Siouxland
500 11th St
Sioux City, IA
(712) 233-1298
FAX (712) 233-1123

KANSAS
Association of Kansas Hospices

Donna Bales
Executive Director
1901 University
Wichita, KS 67213
(316) 263-6380
FAX (316) 263-6542

KENTUCKY
Kentucky Association of Hospices

Susan Hunt
President
c/o Community Hospice
1538 Central Ave
Ashland, KY 41101
(606) 329-1890
FAX (606) 329-0018

LOUISIANA
Louisiana Hospice Organization

Tanya Schreiber
President
c/o Hospice of South Louisiana
210 Mystic Blvd
Houma, LA 70360-2762
(504) 851-4273
FAX (504) 872-6543

MAINE
Maine Hospice Council
Kandyce Powell
Executive Director
16 Winthrop St
Augusta, ME 04330
(207) 626-0651
FAX (207) 626-0651

MARYLAND
Hospice Network of Maryland

Susan Riggs

Executive Director
5820 Southwestern Blvd.
Baltimore, MD 21227
(410) 242-1075
FAX (410) 247-4426

MASSACHUSETTS
Hospice Federation of Massachusetts

Diane Stringer
President
c/o Hospice of the North Shore
10 Elm St
Danvers, MA 01923-2848
(508) 774-7566
FAX (508) 774-4389

MICHIGAN
Michigan Hospice Organization

Sue Wierengo
Executive Director
900 Third Street
Muskegon, MI 49440
(616) 722-2257
FAX (616) 722-7898

MINNESOTA
Minnesota Hospice Organization

Daniel T Holst
Executive Director
Iris Park Place, Suite 36
1885 University Ave W
St. Paul, MN 55104-3403
(612) 659-0423
FAX (612) 659-0514

MISSISSIPPI
Mississippi Hospice Organization

John C Fletcher

President
c/o Hospice of Central Mississippi
2600 Insurance Ctr Dr
Suite B120
Jackson, MS 39216
(601) 366-9811
FAX (601) 981-0150

MISSOURI
Missouri Hospice Organization

Cindy Newport
Executive Director
1625 W 92nd St
Kansas City, MO 64114
(816) 363-2600
FAX (816) 523-0068

MONTANA
Montana Hospice Organization

Julia A Jardine
President
c/o Gateway Hospice
504 S 13th St
Livingston, MT 59047-3727
(406) 222-5030
FAX (406) 222-5099

NEBRASKA
Nebraska Hospice Organization

Marcia Cederdahl
President
c/o Hospice Care of Nebraska
1600 S 70th St, Suite 201
Lincoln, NE 68509
(402) 488-1363
FAX (402) 488-5976

NEVADA
Hospice Association of Nevada

Susan Drongowski
President
c/o Nathan Adelson Hospice
4141 S Swenson St
Las Vegas, NV 89119-6718
(702) 733-0320
FAX (702) 731-5531

NEW HAMPSHIRE
New Hampshire Hospice Organization

Marie Kirn
Executive Director
PO Box 638
Concord, NH 03302-0638
1-(800) 639-8594

NEW JERSEY
New Jersey Hospice Organization

Donald L Pendley
Executive Director
175 Glenside Ave
Scotch Plains, NJ 07076
(908) 233-0060
FAX (908) 233-1630

NEW MEXICO
New Mexico Hospice Association

Ann R Gerber
President
c/o The Hospice Center
1422 Paseo de Peralta
Santa Fe, NM 87501
(505) 988-2211
FAX (505) 986-1833

NEW YORK
New York State Hospice Assoc.

Amber B Jones
Executive Director
21 Aviation Rd, Suite 9
Albany, NY 12205
(518) 446-1483
FAX (518) 446-1484

NORTH CAROLINA
Hospice for the Carolinas

Judi Lund Person
Executive Director
400 Oberlin Rd, Suite 300
Raleigh, NC 27605
(919) 829-9588
FAX (919) 829-1383

NORTH DAKOTA
North Dakota Hospice Org.

Terry L Mahar
President
c/o United Hospice
PO Box 6002, 1200 S Columbia
Grand Forks, ND 58206-6002
(701) 780-5258
FAX (701) 783-5849

OHIO
Ohio Hospice Organization

Bernice Wilson
Executive Director
2400 Briggs Rd
Columbus, OH 43223
(614) 274-9513
FAX (614) 274-6357

OKLAHOMA
Oklahoma State Hospice Association

Cathie Sales
President

c/o Russell-Murray Hospice
PO Box 1423, 117 N Bickford
El Reno, OK 73036
(405) 262-3088
FAX (405) 262-6932

OREGON
Oregon Hospice Association

Ann Jackson
Executive Director
PO Box 10796
Portland, OR 97210
(503) 228-2104
FAX (503) 222-4907

PENNSYLVANIA
Pennsylvania Hospice Network

Denise S. Schlegel
Executive Director
PO Box 60636
Harrisburg, PA 17106-0636
(717) 682-3372
FAX (717) 671-3712

PUERTO RICO
Puerto Rico Home Health and Hospice Association

Emerita Vazquez
President
c/o Puerto Rico Home Care and Hospice Association
Apartado 954
Atjuntas, PR 00601
(809) 829-7710
FAX (809) 829-1372

RHODE ISLAND
Hospice Care of Rhode Island

David Rehm
Contact Person

169 George St
Pawtucket, RI 02860-3868
(401) 727-7070

SOUTH CAROLINA
Hospice for the Carolinas

Tambra Medley
Executive Director
241 Lake Summit Dr
Chapin, SC 29036
(803) 345-0274
FAX (803) 345-0754

SOUTH DAKOTA
South Dakota Hospice Organization

Sandy Young
President
c/o Sioux Valley Hospital Hospice
1100 S Euclid Ave
Sioux Falls, SD 57117-5039
(605) 333-4440
FAX (605) 333-1576

TENNESSEE
Tennessee Hospice Organization

Sarah Gorodezky
President
c/o Alive Hospice
PO Box 23588
Nashville, TN 37202-3588
(615) 327-1085
FAX (615) 327-1166

TEXAS
Texas Hospice Organization

Larry Farrow
Executive Director
3724 Jefferson #318

Austin, TX 78734
(512) 454-1247

UTAH
Utah Hospice Organization

Carma Mark
President
c/o Hospice of IHC
2250 South 1300, Suite A
Salt Lake City, UT 84119
(801) 977-9900
FAX (801) 977-9956

VERMONT
Hospice Council of Vermont

Virginia L. Fry
Executive Director
52 State Street
Montpelier, VT 05602
(802) 229-0579

VIRGINIA
Virginia Association for Hospice
Beth Amos
Executive Director
PO Box 34765
Richmond, VA 23234
(804) 743-7644
FAX (804) 743-7941

WASHINGTON
Washington State Hospice Organization

Tom Halazon
President
c/o Tri-Cities Chaplaincy
7525 W Deschutes Pl, Suite 2A
Kennewick, WA 99336-7747
(509) 783-7416
FAX (509) 735-7850

WEST VIRGINIA
Hospice Council of West Virginia

Malene Smith Davis
President
c/o Hospice Care Corporation
PO Box 229
Kingwood, WV 26537
(304) 329-1161
FAX (304) 329-3285

WISCONSIN
Wisconsin Hospice Organization

Jeanne Bruce
Executive Director
PO Box 366
White Water, WI 53910
(414) 473-7847
FAX (414) 473-7867

WYOMING
Wyoming Hospice Organization

Sue Carrole Klus
President
1023 Teewinot Cir
Gillette, WY 82716-4135
(307) 682-6122

Q: Are there any other agencies that might be able to help me?

Yes. See the list of useful addresses that follows.

Academy of Hospice Nurses
Marilyn Harton
President
32478 Dunford Rd
Farmington Hills, MI 48334
(810) 489-0937
FAX (810) 591-8356

Academy of Hospice Physicians *see* American Academy of
Hospice and Palliative Medicine

*AIDS and Persons with Developmental Disabilities: The Legal
Perspective*
     American Bar Association
     Center on Children and the Law
     1800 M Street NW
     Washington, D.C. 20036
     (202) 331-2200

AIDS National Interfaith Network (ANIN)
     Ken Smith
     Executive Director
     110 Maryland Avenue NE, Suite 504
     Washington, D.C. 20002
     (202) 546-0807
     FAX (202) 546-5103

Alzheimer's Disease & Related Disorders Association, Inc.
     919 North Michigan Avenue
     Chicago, IL 60611
     1-(800) 621-0379
     1-(800) 572-6037 (Illinois residents)

Alzheimer's Disease Education & Referrals
     1-(800) 438-4380

American Academy of Hospice and Palliative Medicine
     Dale C. Smith
     Executive Director
     PO Box 14288
     Gainesville, FL 32604-2288
     (352) 377-8900
     FAX (352) 371-2349

American Association of Retired People (AARP)
     601 E Street NW B5640
     Washington, D.C. 20049
     (202) 434-2277

also from AARP
Path for the Caregiver
(Stock No. D1297)

AARP Fulfillment
1909 K Street NW
Washington, D.C. 22049

The American Institute of Life-Threatening Illness and Loss
  (A Division of The Foundation of Thanatology)
Dr. Austin H. Kutscher, President
Columbia-Presbyterian Medical Ctr
630 West 168th Street
New York, NY 10032
(212) 928-2066 or (914) 779-4877 or (718) 601-4453
FAX (914) 793-0813 or (718) 549-7219

American Journal of Hospice and Palliative Care (published bimonthly)
  470 Boston Post Road
  Weston, MA 02193
  (617) 899-2702

ARCH (Access to Respite Care and Help)
  800 Eastowne Dr, Suite 105
  Chapel Hill, NC 27514
  1-(800) 473-1727 (Hotline)

Association for Death Education and Counseling
  Suzanne Berry
  Executive Director
  638 Prospect Avenue
  Hartford, CT 06105-4298
  (203) 586-7503
  FAX (203) 586-7550

Association of Nurses in AIDS Care (ANAC)
  1555 Connecticut Avenue NW, Suite 200
  Washington, D.C. 20036
  (202) 462-1038

Candlelighters Childhood Cancer Foundation
   7910 Woodmont Ave., Suite 460
   Bethesda, MD 20814
   1-(800) 366-2223

Children's Hospice International, Inc. (CHI)
   1850 M Street NW, Suite 900
   Washington, D.C. 20036
   1-(800) 242-4453
   (703) 684-0330
   FAX (703) 684-0226

Choice in Dying, Inc. (formerly Concern for Dying and Society
for the Right to Die)
   200 Varick Street
   New York, NY 10014
   (212) 366-5540
   FAX (212) 366-5337

Family AIDS Network
   (616) 451-2361

Family Services of America
   11700 West Lake Park Drive
   Milwaukee, WI 53224
   (414) 359-2111

Help Children Cope with Loss
   Grief Resources Foundation
   PO Box 28551
   Dallas, TX 75228

Hospice Association of America/NAHC (National Association
for Home Care)
   519 C Street NE
   Washington, D.C. 20002-5809
   (202) 546-4759

Hospice Education Institute
   Michael J. Galazka

Executive Director
170 Westbrook Road
Essex, CT 06426-1511
(860) 767-1620
1-(800) 331-1620

Hospice Foundation of America
David Abrams
Vice President
777 17th Street, Suite 401
Miami Beach, FL 33139
(305) 538-9272
FAX (305) 538-0092

The Hospice Journal: Physical, Psychosocial and Pastoral Care of the Dying (published quarterly; official journal of the NHO)
The Haworth Press, Inc.
10 Alice Street.
Binghamton, NY 13904-1580
(607) 722-5857

Hospice Nurses Association
Madalon Amenta
Executive Director
5512 Nothumberland Street
Pittsburgh, PA 15217-1131
(412) 687-3231
FAX (412) 687-9095

International Hospice Institute
Jean Bergaust
Executive Director
1275 K Street NW, 10th Floor
Washington, D.C. 20005
(202) 842-1600
FAX (202) 682-2127

Journal of Palliative Care
  Electa Baril
  Assistant Editor
  110 Pine Avenue West
  Montreal, Canada H2W 1R7

National AIDS Hotline
  (24-hour, toll-free service providing confidential information, referrals, educational material.)
  1-(800) 342-AIDS
  Servicio en Español: 1-(800) 344-7432
  TTY/TDD for Hearing Impaired: 1-(800) 243-7889

National AIDS Information Clearing House
  PO Box 6003
  Rockville, MD 20850
  1-(800) 458-5231

National Association of People with AIDS
  Jillian M. Mackin
  Membership Marketing
  1413 K Street NW, 8th Floor
  Washington, DC 20005
  (202) 898-0414
  FAX (202) 898-0435

National Consumers League
  Linda F. Golodner
  Executive Director
  815 Fifteenth Street, NW
  Suite 516
  Washington, D.C. 20005
  (202) 639-8140

National Funeral Directors Assoc.
  Robert E. Harden
  Executive Director
  11121 West Oklahoma Avenue
  Milwaukee, WI 53227-4096

(414) 541-2500
FAX (414) 541-1909
1-(800) 228-6332

National Hospice Organization (NHO)
Hospice (journal published quarterly by the NHO)
1901 North Moore Street
Suite 901
Arlington, VA 22209
(703) 243-5900
FAX (703) 525-5762
Hospice Helpline: 1-(800) 658-8898

National Institute for Jewish Hospice
247 East Tahquitz Canyon Way
Suite 21
Palm Springs, CA 92263
(619) 323-3555
1-(800) 446-4448

Native American AIDS Hotline
1-(800) 283-2437

Nurse Healers—Professional Associates, Inc.
PO Box 444
Allison Park, PA 15101-0444
(412) 355-8476
(Write for contact person in your area.)

Oncology Nursing Society
Pearl Moore
Executive Director
501 Holiday Drive
Pittsburgh, PA 15220-2749
(412) 921-7373
FAX (412) 921-6565

Oncology Nursing Society
AIDS/HIV Special Interest Group (SIG)
501 Holiday Drive

Pittsburgh, PA 15220-2749
(412) 921-7373
FAX (412) 921-6565

Pediatric AIDS Foundation (PAF)
1311 Colorado Avenue
Santa Monica, CA 90404
(310) 395-9051
1-(800) 488-5000

Physician's Association for AIDS Care
Mabrey R. Whigham, III
Membership Services Director
10940 Wilshire Blvd, Suite 1600
Los Angeles, CA 90024
(312) 222-1326
FAX (312) 222-0329

THANATOS: A Realistic Journal Concerning Dying, Death and Bereavement (published quarterly by the Florida Funeral Director Services)
PO Box 6009
Tallahassee, FL 32314-9990
(904) 224-1969

Theos Foundation
International Headquarters
322 Blvd of the Allies, Suite 105
Pittsburgh, PA 15222
(412) 471-7779
FAX (412) 471-7782

Visiting Nurse Association of America
Sherril Banks
Information Specialist
3801 East Florida, Suite 900
Denver, CO 80210
(303) 753-0218
FAX (303) 753-0258

Q: Can you suggest some books for me to read?

Suggested Reading

American Association of Retired People. *Path for the Caregiver* (Stock #D1297). AARP Fulfillment, 1609 K Street NW, Washington, DC 22049.

American Bar Association. *AIDS and Persons with Developmental Disabilities: The Legal Perspective*. Washington, DC, 1990.

American Journal of Hospice and Palliative Care. Weston, MA. Bimonthly.

Becker, Ernest. *The Denial of Death*. New York: Free Press, 1985.

Beresford, Larry. *The Hospice Handbook*. Boston, MA: Little, Brown & Co., 1993.

Blunt, Kathie, and Scalzo, Lilah. *Someone Special Died*. Loma Linda, CA: Loma Linda Hospice, 1990.

Buckingham, Robert W. *Among Friends: Hospice Care for the Person with AIDS*. Amherst, NY: Prometheus Books, 1992.

Coleman, Barbara. *A Consumer Guide to Hospice Care*. Washington, DC: National Consumers League, Revised 1990.

Cousins, Norman. *The Healing Heart*. New York: Norton Co., 1983.

Dane, Barbara O., and Levin, Carol, eds., *AIDS and the New Orphans*. Westport, CT: Auburn House, 1994.

Geballe, Shelley, et al., eds., *The Forgotten Children of the AIDS Epidemic*. New Haven, CT: Yale University Press, 1995.

Hospice. Arlington, VA: National Hospice Organization (NHO). Quarterly.

——. Special Pediatric Issue, funded by the Loewen Children's Foundation (November 1995), 6(5).

The Hospice Journal: Physical, Psychosocial and Pastoral Care of the Dying. Binghamton, NY: The Haworth Press, Inc. Quarterly.

Journal of Palliative Care. Montreal, Canada.

Kübler-Ross, Elisabeth. *Living with Death and Dying*. New York: Macmillan, 1981.

——. *On Death and Dying*. New York: Macmillan, 1969.

——. *Questions and Answers on Death and Dying*. New York: Macmillan, 1974.

———. *To Live Until We Say Good-Bye.* Englewood Cliffs, NJ: Prentice-Hall, 1978.

Kushner, Harold S. *When Bad Things Happen To Good People.* New York: Avon, 1982.

Levin, Carol, and Stein, Gary L. *Orphans of the HIV Epidemic.* New York: The Orphan Project, 1994.

Levine, Stephen. *Who Dies? An Investigation of Conscious Living and Dying.* New York: Anchor Press/Doubleday, 1982.

Lewis, C. S. *A Grief Observed.* New York: Bantam Books, Inc., 1976.

MacDonald, N. "The Hospice Movement: An Oncologist's Viewpoint." *CA—A Cancer Journal for Clinicians* (July-August 1984) 31(4).

Mount, Balfour. *Sightings.* Downers Grove, IL: InterVarsity Press, 1983.

Munley, Anne G. *The Hospice Alternative.* New York: Basic Books, Inc., 1983.

National Hospice Organization. *Alternative Care Programs in Hospice.* Arlington, VA: NHO Alternative Care Task Force, 1991.

———. *Resource Manual for Providing Hospice Care to People Living with AIDS.* Arlington, VA: NHO 1994-1995 AIDS Resource Committee, 1996.

Rando, Therese A. *Loss and Anticipatory Grief.* New York: Free Press, 1986.

Reynolds, Jeffrey L., writer and editor. *Reclaiming Lost Voices: Children Orphaned by HIV/AIDS in Suburbia.* Huntington Station, NY: Long Island Association for AIDS Care, Inc. (LIAAC), August, 1995.

Riemer, Jack. *Jewish Reflections on Death.* New York: Schocken Books, 1987.

Rosen, Elliot J. *Families Facing Death.* New York: Free Press [Lexington Books], 1990.

Sankar, Andrea. *Dying at Home.* Baltimore, MD: The Johns Hopkins University Press, 1991.

Saunders, Cicely. "Death, Dying and the Hospice Movement," in *Oxford Companion to Medicine.* Oxford: Oxford University Press, 1986.

———. *The Management of Terminal Disease.* London: Edward Arnold, 1986.

Schaefer, Dan, and Lyons, Christine. *How Do We Tell The Children?* New York: Newmarket Press, 1986.

Stoddard, Sandol. *The Hospice Movement: a better way of caring for the dying* (Rev ed.). New York: Random House, Inc. (Vintage Press), 1992.

THANATOS: A Realistic Journal Concerning Dying, Death and Bereavement. Tallahassee, FL. Quarterly.

Viorst, Judith. *Necessary Losses.* New York: Simon and Schuster, 1986.

Worden, William J. *Grief Counseling and Grief Therapy.* New York: Springer, 1982.

APPENDIX A
FORMS

CONTENTS

Reference for all Figures: Long Island Foundation for Hospice
Care and Research, Inc., *Hospice Operations Manual* (Hempstead,
NY: 1990).

CONTROLLED DRUG DISPOSAL RECORD

Patient _____

Physician _____

Drug Name _____

    Form _____

    Strength _____

Date Prescribed _____

Date Discontinued _____

Amount Remaining _____

Amount Destroyed _____

This drug was destroyed today according to the Policies and Procedures

of Hospice.

Hospice Nurse _____

Witness _____

Date _____

Figure 1. Controlled Drug Disposal Record

HOSPICE INFORMED CONSENT FORM

WE, THE PATIENT AND CAREGIVER, REQUEST ADMISSION TO THE HOSPICE PROGRAM
AND UNDERSTAND AND AGREE TO THE FOLLOWING CONDITIONS:

Introduction: We understand that the Hospice Program is palliative, not
curative, in its goals. The program emphasizes the identification and
the relief of symptoms such as pain and physical discomfort and
addresses the spiritual needs and the emotional stress which the Patient
and Family may experience and which may accompany the life-threatening
illness for which the Patient is being admitted.

_____ As the Patient, I ask that my Family member(s) or Significant
        Other(s) respect my choice of Hospice care and, insofar as they
        are able, that they fulfill the role of Primary Caregiver for me.

_____ As the Family member(s) or Significant Other(s), I/we understand
        the role of Primary Caregiver and, insofar as I/we are able,
        pledge to undertake that role with the training and support of the
        Hospice Interdisciplinary Team.

Caregiver: We understand that Hospice services are not intended to take
the place of care by Family members or others who are important to the
Patient, but rather, to instruct and aid them in the care of the
Patient. With the help of HOSPICE, the person designated as "Caregiver"
will provide around-the-clock care to the Patient at home. If twenty-
four (24) hour care is not available, the Caregiver will arrange for
another to provide it. The "Caregiver" also will participate in
decisions about the care provided to the Patient at home and/or in the
inpatient setting.

Home Care: We understand that Home Care is the main focus of the Hospice
program. Services are provided in the patient's place of residence by an
Interdisciplinary Team of Hospice Staff and Volunteers, through
scheduled visits. These services are available both on a scheduled basis
and as needed. Emergency consultation and visits are available twenty-
four (24) hours a day, seven (7) days a week. In a medical crisis,
Hospice may provide around-the-clock care for a few days in order to
allow the Patient to stay at home.

Inpatient Care: We understand that if it is determined necessary by
Hospice and the Patient's Attending Physician, the Patient can receive
short-term care in an inpatient facility. Admission to the inpatient
setting will be arranged if there is a continuing presence of symptoms
that fail to yield to home care management. Other reasons may be
determined on an individual basis.

We understand that the inpatient care will be provided in a HOSPICE
contracted hospital. If the patient is admitted to a non-contract
hospital, the patient/family will be responsible for costs incurred and

Figure 2. Hospice Informed Consent Form (Page 1)

HOSPICE will not be responsible for any costs incurred in this situation.

We understand that if, after admission to the inpatient setting, the Hospice Interdisciplinary Team decides there is no longer need for Hospice inpatient care, the Patient will be discharged from the inpatient setting. The Hospice Staff will provide assistance to us in making discharge plans.

Follow-up Care for Families: We understand that the "Caregiver" and others who are part of the Patient's Family, or who are important to the Patient, may choose to participate in the Hospice Bereavement Program. Services designed for Family members and others include individual counseling, group support, help with practical matters, and social events.

Choice of Care: We understand that the patient and the Family may give input and are considered to be a part of the Hospice Interdisciplinary Team. We understand that we will have a choice about the care provided to us. We may review the Plan of Care that guides Hospice services and, if we desire, may refuse a particular treatment or service offered.

We further understand that some medical services or procedures (such as advanced cardiac life supports or respirators) may not be provided by Hospice. We are aware that the subject of resuscitation should be discussed by us and our Physician prior to Hospice acceptance. Other services are provided only if they are determined by our Physician to be necessary for the comfort of the Patient.

Records: We authorize HOSPICE to obtain copies of medical and billing records and to keep records which include necessary personal information about the Patient's medical condition, Family and finances during the time in which we are under the care of the HOSPICE Program.

We permit the release of necessary information and medical records to or from any appropriate agency or medical person/physician as required, to assure coordination and continuity of care and as necessary for reimbursement. Except as required for patient care, reimbursement, or quality control, such records will not be released to persons outside HOSPICE without our written consent.

Financial Responsibility: The estimated cost and expected reimbursement of Hospice care has been explained to us. We have read the attached explanation regarding the benefits, provisions, and scope of services to be offered us. We understand that we are responsible for payment for those services not covered by insurance unless other arrangements for payment have been made. We have been given a chance to discuss our financial needs with a representative of HOSPICE. We understand that we are required to meet these financial responsibilities to the extent possible, and that the Patient's acceptance into the Hospice Program will be determined on an individual basis.

Figure 2. Hospice Informed Consent Form (Page 2)

Withdrawal/Discharge: We accept the conditions of HOSPICE as described, understanding that we may choose not to remain in the program and that Hospice may discharge us from the program if Hospice care is no longer appropriate. This means there will be no further liability to us or to HOSPICE. We understand, however, that we may request to be readmitted at a later date.

We have been able to discuss the above conditions with a member of the HOSPICE staff and have had our questions answered to our satisfaction.

Signature of Patient or Legal Guardian   Date

Name of Patient or Legal Guardian   (If applicable): Address and Telephone
(Please print)   of Legal Guardian:

_____

_____

(   ) _____

Signature of Primary Caregiver   Date

Name of Primary Caregiver (Please print) Relationship of Primary Caregiver to
                                          Patient

                                          Address and Telephone Number of
                                          Primary Caregiver, if different from
                                          that of Patient:

_____

_____

(   ) _____

Signature of Hospice Representative   Date

Name of Hospice Representative (Please print)   Date

Figure 2. Hospice Informed Consent Form (Page 3)

HOSPICE

STATEMENT PROHIBITING REDISCLOSURE

OF CONFIDENTIAL INFORMATION

_____   _____

PATIENT'S NAME   DATE

_____

TO WHOM INFORMATION DISCLOSED

"This information has been disclosed to you from confidential records
which are protected by state law. State law prohibits you from making
any further disclosure of this information without the specific written
consent of the person to whom it pertains, or as otherwise permitted by
law. Any unauthorized further disclosure in violation of state law may
result in a fine or jail sentence or both. A general authorization for
the release of medical or other information is NOT sufficient
authorization for further disclosure."

                              _____

                                      Signature

_Figure 3. Hospice Statement Prohibiting Redisclosure of Confidential
Information_

<Attending Physician>, M.D.
123 4th Street
Maintown, New York 00000

Dear Dr. _____:

_____<Patient's Name>_____ has been admitted as a Hospice patient.
We are in the process of formulating a Plan of Care for this patient.
Since you have been providing services to him/her, your input into this
plan is necessary to make it complete. Therefore, we request that the
following be sent to the Hospice office, so that it can be included in
the patient's record:

1.   Copy of Assessment,

2.   Plan of Care, and

3.   Summary of Services Provided.

Enclosed is a copy of the Patient's Consent, which gives us permission
to have access to their health care records. After we receive the above
information, we will notify you of the time and place of the
interdisciplinary team meeting for this patient. We welcome you and
encourage you to attend.

These steps will hopefully serve to coordinate our efforts and thus help
us to deliver the best of care to our patients. Please call at any time
with questions, concerns, and changes in the patient's condition.

Your cooperation and support are most appreciated.

Sincerely yours,

Patient Care Coordinator

Enclosure

Figure 4. Letter from Hospice to New Patient's Attending Physician

ATTENDING PHYSICIAN AUTHORIZATION

PHYSICIAN _____   PATIENT _____

ADDRESS _____

DATE OF REFERRAL _____

I give my consent for the above named Patient to be admitted to the
Hospice Program of Care based upon my diagnosis that this patient is
suffering from a chronic progressive illness with a <u>life expectancy of
six (6) months or less</u>.

I request the <u>Hospice Physician to work with me</u> in the care of my
Patient. I understand that the Hospice Physician gives medical direction
to the Hospice patient care team, that he/she is available as a
consultant to me, and as indicated by the Hospice Plan of Care, that
<u>he/she provides direct symptom control services to the patient,
including inpatient, outpatient, and home care visits</u>. I request that
the Hospice Physician <u>see my patient</u> in order to appropriately develop
the individual Plan of Care and give medical direction to the Hospice
Interdisciplinary Team.

I authorize the Hospice Physician to admit my Patient to Hospice
inpatient care, upon consent of the patient and family, should such
inpatient care be needed for the control of pain, symptoms, or for the
relief of the primary caregiver. I UNDERSTAND THAT I WILL BE CONSULTED
PRIOR TO ANY ADMISSION TO INPATIENT CARE UNLESS I AM NOT AVAILABLE AND
THE NEED FOR ADMISSION IS SEVERE. I understand that I may obtain
privileges to write orders for my Patient's care on the unit by going
through the credentialing process established by the inpatient facility,
and that these orders will be consistent with the above Patient's
Hospice Plan of Care.

I authorize the Hospice Interdisciplinary Team to teach the
Patient/Family to administer medications.

I understand that I continue to be this Patient's Primary/Attending
Physician.

I understand that I will be consulted about the Hospice Plan of Care for
this Patient, that I will be welcome at all Interdisciplinary Team
conferences concerning this Patient, that I am considered to be a member
of that Interdisciplinary Team, and that Care Progress Summaries will be
forwarded to me on a regular basis.

I understand that the Hospice Program of Care is <u>palliative, not
curative</u> in its goals and techniques, focusing on the alleviation of
pain and other symptoms and not employing medical and surgical heroic
measures or artificial life support systems.

Figure 5. Attending Physician Authorization (Page 1)

I understand that Hospice services are primarily designed to be
delivered in Patients' own homes, and that institutional care is used
for short stays, primarily for intensive pain and symptom control, and
directed toward assisting the Family and Patient to be strong enough
physically and emotionally to be cared for at home, if at all possible.

I understand that Admission to the Hospice Program is dependent upon the
Informed Consent of the Patient/Family and upon their meeting the
Admission Criteria of the Program.

PLEASE INDICATE THE EXTENT TO WHICH YOU WOULD LIKE THE HOSPICE PHYSICIAN
TO BE INVOLVED IN THE DIRECT CARE OF THIS PATIENT: (CHOOSE ONE)

_____ The Hospice Physician may write medication or treatment orders and
arrange for medical supplies, paramedical services, _and admission
to the inpatient unit_ at his/her discretion, and keep me informed
through routine progress reports.

_____ I wish to be contacted directly should the need arise for a change
in or addition to current care. However, if I am not immediately
available, the Hospice Physician may write initial orders, subject
to my later confirmation and based on the Hospice Plan of Care.

PLEASE INDICATE YOUR PREFERENCE REGARDING DEATH CERTIFICATE SHOULD THIS
PATIENT DIE AT HOME OR IN THE INPATIENT UNIT: (CHOOSE ONE)

_____ I will sign the Death Certificate.

_____ The Hospice Physician may sign the Death Certificate.

PLEASE SIGN AND RETURN ONE COPY IN THE ENCLOSED ENVELOPE

PHYSICIAN'S SIGNATURE _____ DATE _____

NOTE: For Medicare Patients, must be signed no later than two (2) days
after Hospice care is initiated.

Figure 5. Attending Physician Authorization (Page 2)

The patient, _____,
                      -(Name)

and the patient's next of kin, or primary caregiver,

_____,
      (Name)   (Relationship)

agree to:

___ Provide the Hospice Team with complete medical history and
    information necessary for the planning and delivery of appropriate
    care.

___ Discuss needs and preferences with the Hospice Team members.

___ Participate in the developing of a Plan of Care.

___ Report _immediately_ to the Hospice staff any changes in the
    condition of the patient which will affect the Plan of Care.
    (Hospice staff may be contacted twenty-four (24) hours a day.)

___ Follow the policy and procedure of the Hospice in handling and
    caring for drugs and/or equipment supplied by the Hospice.

___ Notify Hospice staff _immediately_ of any decision to seek or obtain
    treatment or services not included in the Hospice Plan of Care.

I understand that HOSPICE will not be financially responsible for any
hospitalization not authorized by Hospice and not in the Hospice Plan of
Care. It is agreed that should such unauthorized hospitalization occur,
the financial obligation will be that of the patient/family.

I understand that I may choose care other than Hospice at any time. Such
a choice will automatically relieve HOSPICE of any responsibility for
further provision of care.

Patient: _____
              (Signature)   (Date)

Figure 6. Patient/Family Consent Form (Prior to Hospice Admission)

<u>DNR DOCUMENTATION SHEET #1</u>
<u>ADULT PATIENT WITH CAPACITY</u>
<u>WRITTEN CONSENT</u>

I, _____, hereby consent to my attending
physician issuing a Do Not Resuscitate Order, in the event I suffer
cardiac or respiratory arrest subject to the following conditions, if
any: _____

_____

I have been advised by my attending physician regarding information
about diagnosis and prognosis, the range of available resuscitation
measures, the reasonable foreseeable risks and benefits of CPR for me
and the consequences of a DNR order.

                        Patient _____
                                            (Signature)

                              <u>WITNESSES</u>

Witness 1 _____   Witness 2 _____
                (Signature)   (Signature)

Name _____   Name _____
                (Print)   (Print)

Relationship_____   Relationship_____
Age _____   Age _____
Date _____   Date _____

Indicate action taken (check one):
_____ Do Not Resuscitate Order Issued For _____
                                            Patient's Name

                                       _____
                                       Physician's Signature

                                       _____
                                       Date

_____ Patient transferred to another attending Physician
_____ Referred to dispute mediation system

Figure 7. DNR Documentation Sheet No. 1: Adult Patient with Capacity—
Written Consent

DNR DOCUMENTATION SHEET #2

ADULT PATIENT WITH CAPACITY

ORAL CONSENT

Directions: This Documentation Sheet sets forth in consecutive order the steps that must be followed before writing a DNR order for an ADULT patient with CAPACITY. When completed, this Sheet must be placed in the patient's medical record.

The ATTENDING PHYSICIAN must obtain the oral consent of the patient to a DNR order. Oral consent must be given in the presence of a physician on staff at the Hospice and a witness.

Attending Physician's Statement

The patient has expressed orally in my presence, or in the presence of another physician on staff at the hospital (indicate name: _____ _____), the decision to consent to a DNR order. I have provided to the patient information about his/her diagnosis and prognosis, the reasonably foreseeable risks and benefits of cardiopulmonary resuscitation for him/her, and the consequences of a DNR order. I have determined that the patient has the ability to understand and appreciate the nature and consequences of a DNR order, including the benefits and disadvantages, and to reach an informed decision.

_____
Signature

_____
Date

Witness' Statement

The patient has expressed orally in my presence the decision to consent to a DNR order.

_____
Signature

_____
Print Name

_____
Title/Relationship to Patient

_____
Date

Figure 8. DNR Documentation Sheet No. 2: Adult Patient with Capacity—Oral Consent

<u>DNR DOCUMENTATION SHEET #3</u>

<u>ADULT PATIENT WITHOUT CAPACITY</u>

<u>AND WITH A SURROGATE</u>

<u>Determination of Capacity</u>

I have examined _____ and have determined,
to a reasonable degree of medical certainty, that he/she lacks the
ability to understand and appreciate the nature and consequences of a
DNR order, including the benefits and disadvantages, and to reach an
informed decision. In my opinion, the cause of the patient's incapacity
is _____ and its extent
and probable duration are _____
_____.

Date: _____ Attending Physician: _____

<u>Concurring Physician's Statement</u>

I have personally examined _____ and have
determined, to a reasonable degree of medical certainty, that he/she
lacks the ability to understand and appreciate the nature and
consequences of a DNR order, including the benefits and disadvantages,
and to reach an informed decision. In my opinion, the cause of the
patient's incapacity is _____
and its extent and probable duration are _____
_____.

Date: _____ Concurring Physician: _____

<u>Determination of Surrogate</u>

To the best of my knowledge, the surrogate is:

Date: _____ Surrogate: _____
                                              (Name)

                          Relationship to Patient _____

                          Attending Physician _____

*Figure 9. DNR Documentation Sheet No. 3: Adult Patient without Capacity—
and with a Surrogate*

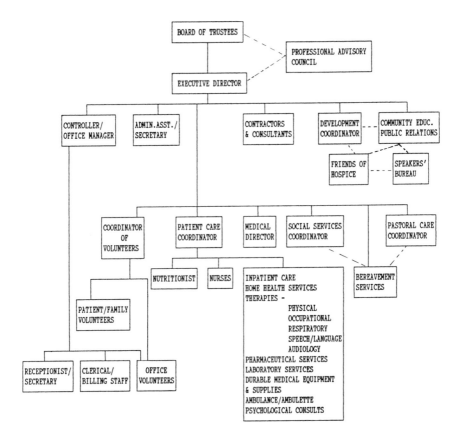

Figure 10. Organizational Chart by Employment and Supervision: Independent Community-Based Hospice (Not-for-Profit)

Service/Items*	Hospice	Hospital	Home Health
Medications to be used at home for control of pain and other symptoms	Yes	No	No
Services covered even if the patient is not home bound	Yes	No	No
Deductible waived	Yes	No	Yes
Inpatient respite care to provide rest for home caregivers	Yes	No	No
Continuous care at home during periods of crisis	Yes	No	No
Counseling services at home for both the patient and family	Yes	No	No
Bereavement counseling	Yes	No	No
Trained volunteers must be available	Yes	No	No
Inpatient unit must provide specialized Hospice care	Yes	No	—
Care available to residents in nursing homes	Yes	No	No

*No deductibles, no co-insurance required, with the exception of a 5% co-payment for medications and respite care.

Figure 11. The Hospice Benefit and Other Medicare Benefits

MEDICARE HOSPICE BENEFITS ELECTION

As a Medicare Part A Beneficiary, I request that the Hospice Benefit be made available to me through HOSPICE. I understand that Hospice care is palliative, not curative as it relates to the illness for which I am being admitted. I also understand that while this election is in force, Medicare will make payments for care related to this illness only to the Physician designated below and to Hospice, and that services related to this illness provided by hospitals, home health agencies, nursing homes, and any other company or agency will not be reimbursed by Medicare unless specifically ordered and authorized by Hospice. I understand that services not related to this illness continue to be covered by Medicare along with Hospice benefits. I understand that I may revoke this election at any time and thereby restore my usual Medicare Benefits.

WE ACKNOWLEDGE THAT WE HAVE BEEN GIVEN AMPLE OPPORTUNITY TO ASK ANY AND ALL QUESTIONS WE HAVE CONCERNING THE HOSPICE PROGRAM OF CARE. FOR MEDICARE PURPOSES, WE ACKNOWLEDGE WE HAVE READ AND AGREE TO THE HOSPICE BENEFITS ELECTION PRINTED ABOVE.

Patient or Representative

Relationship of above Representative to Patient

Date

Witness

Admission Date

Effective Date of Election

Other Family Member

Person identified by the Patient as being Family or Significant Other or who is the Legally Responsible Person for this Patient.

Address

Telephone

Physician Designated by the Patient as Attending Physician (please print full name).

Address

Telephone

Figure 12. Medicare Hospice Benefits Election (Page 1)

(for office use only)

ELECTION FOR BENEFIT PERIOD: 1   2   3   4   (Circle one)

REVOCATION DATES, if applicable: _____

                                         _____

Original to Medical Records
2nd copy to Billing
3rd copy to Patient

Figure 12. Medicare Hospice Benefits Election (Page 2)

HOSPICE BENEFIT REVOCATION FORM

PATIENT NUMBER _____   ADMIT DATE _____

DIAGNOSIS _____   INSURANCE NUMBER _____

_____   Address/Telephone of Patient:
Patient Name (Please Print)

                                          _____

_____   _____
Date of Birth
                                          (____)_____

_____   Address/Telephone of Attendin
Attending Physician Name (Please print)   Physician:

                                          _____

                                          _____

                                          (____)_____

I, _____, hereby revoke my election to
Hospice Care for the remainder of the current election period.

        Date Election Period Began   _____

        Date of Revocation   _____

        Number of Days Remaining   _____

I understand that I am no longer covered by Medicare for Hospice
services but may resume regular Medicare benefits previously waived.

I understand that I may at any time again elect to receive Hospice
coverage for any other Hospice election period for which I am eligible.

_____   _____
Signature of Patient   Date

_____   _____
Signature of Witness   Date

_____
Name of Witness (Please Print)

Figure 13. Hospice Benefits Revocation Form

REQUEST FOR CHANGE OF DESIGNATED HOSPICE

Patient Name: _____

Medicare Number: _____

I, _____, plan to transfer from

<Name of Hospice> _____ to

<Name of Hospice> _____ .

I understand that I may change Hospice services only once in each
benefit period and retain Medicare Hospice benefits.

        Patient's signature: _____

        Effective date of transfer: _____

- -

<Name of Hospice>

REQUEST FOR CHANGE OF DESIGNATED HOSPICE

Patient Name: _____

Medicare Number: _____

I, _____, plan to transfer from

<Name of Hospice> _____ to

<Name of Hospice> _____ .

I understand that I may change Hospice services only once in each
benefit period and retain Medicare Hospice benefits.

        Patient's signature: _____

        Effective date of transfer: _____

Figure 14. Request for Change of Designated Hospice

OFFICE SUPPORT VOLUNTEER APPLICATION

Name: _____ Phone: (___) _____

Address: _____
                                                    (Zip)
I can work at home: _____ Office: _____ Both: _____

Days and hours available: _____

_____

I would like to help with the following (please check):

Typing, general
  Correspondence   _____
  Statistical reports   _____
  Newsletter   _____
Filing   _____
Stenography/Dictation   _____

Mailings   _____
  Collate/Staple   _____
  Fold   _____
  Address   _____
  Do Copying   _____

Serve on Telephone Squad   _____
Statistical Reports
  Maintain Volunteer Records   _____
  Maintain Patient Records   _____
  Prepare Reports   _____

Accounting
  Assist with Bookkeeping   _____
  Prepare Financial Reports   _____

Help Maintain Mailing List   _____
Serve on Speakers Bureau   _____

Finance
  Serve on Finance Comm.   _____
  Sell tickets for Special
    Events   _____
  Obtain Ads for Annual
    Journal   _____
  Obtain Memberships   _____

Computer Skills   _____
Word Processing Skills   _____

Hospice Library
  Assist in Maintaining Library   _____
  Maintain Press Clipping Book   _____
  Maintain Bulletin Board   _____
Publicity - Assistance with
  Publicity Releases   _____
  TV and Radio Spots   _____
  Newsletter   _____
  Media Mailing Lists   _____
  Media Kits   _____
Miscellaneous
  Do Art Work   _____
  Do Layout Work   _____
  Assist with Proofreading   _____

  Handle Photography   _____
  Work on Special Educational
    Projects   _____

  Provide Entertainment at Meetings
    and Functions   _____

  Work on Special Research
    Projects   _____

  Transcribe Audio Tapes   _____

  Telephone Operator   _____
  Receptionist   _____

  Other (please specify) _____
_____

Special skills or interest (please
attach resume of skills and experience)

Figure 15. Office Support Volunteer Application

VOLUNTEER INTEREST FORM

1. I would like to volunteer my services:

___ Patient/Family Support   ___ Community Education/Speakers' Bureau

___ Fundraising/Grants   ___ Editorial Assistance/Newsletter

___ Computer Skills   ___ Special Events

___ Office Assistance   ___ Other (please specify) _____

_____

Name: _____
                    (PLEASE PRINT)

Home Address: _____
                                                        (Zip Code)

Business/Group Affiliation (if any): _____

Telephone: (___)_____ (___)_____
              Area Code (Day)   Area Code (Evening)

WHAT IS THE BEST DAY/TIME TO CALL YOU? _____
                                        (Days)   (Times)

2. Please put my name on your mailing list. _____

Figure 16. Volunteer Interest Form

Name: _____ Social Security No. _____

Address: _____
                (No. and Street)   (City)   (Zip)

Home phone: ( ) _____ Business phone: ( ) _____

Birthdate _____ Sex _____ Marital Status _____ Religion (optional) _____

Name of spouse _____ Ages of children _____

Driver's License # _____ Expiration date _____

Do you have current car insurance?   YES _____   NO _____

PERSON TO NOTIFY IN CASE OF ACCIDENT OR EMERGENCY:
Name and relationship _____ Phone ( ) _____

Address _____

Family physician _____Physician's Phone ( ) _____

NAMES OF SCHOOLS ATTENDED (Most recent first)	NO./YEARS	GRADUATED (year)	COURSE OR MAJOR
_____	_____	_____	_____
_____	_____	_____	_____
_____	_____	_____	_____

EMPLOYMENT HISTORY: (Most recent first)

NAME OF EMPLOYER	DATES	DESCRIPTION OF WORK
_____	_____	_____
_____	_____	_____
_____	_____	_____

VOLUNTEER HISTORY: (Most recent first)

NAME OF AGENCY OR INSTITUTION	DATES	DESCRIPTION OF WORK
_____	_____	_____
_____	_____	_____
_____	_____	_____

Figure 17. Hospice Volunteer Application (Page 1)

SPECIAL TRAINING   DATES   DESCRIPTION OF TRAINING

_____   _____   _____

_____   _____   _____

_____   _____   _____

PERSONAL HEALTH   ( ) EXCELLENT   ( ) GOOD   ( ) FAIR

PLEASE NOTE ANY PHYSICAL LIMITATIONS _____

Are you on Workers' Compensation or Disability? ____ If Yes, please
explain _____

Have you ever had cancer?
___ Yes, in the past   ___ Yes, currently in treatment   ___ No

Have you experienced any deaths in your family or of those close to you?
         ___ No   ___ Yes
Please specify your relationship to the persons and when they died.
_____

HOSPICE ROLE DESIRED: (Please check as many as desired.)

1)   Direct Involvement with patient/family (please check)
     LISTENING _____   READING _____   HOUSEKEEPING _____
     VISITING _____   DRIVING _____   BABYSITTING _____

2)   Supportive
     CLERICAL _____   SECRETARIAL _____ NEWSLETTER _____
     TELEPHONE WORK _____   PUBLIC SPEAKING _____   ERRANDS _____
     BABYSITTING FOR OTHER VOLUNTEERS TO FREE THEM FOR DIRECT
     PATIENT CARE, ETC. _____

3)   Other _____

TRANSPORTATION:
DO YOU HAVE A CAR YOU COULD USE TO GET TO PATIENTS' HOMES? __ YES __ NO
__ SOMETIMES

HOW FAR FROM YOUR HOME WOULD IT BE FEASIBLE FOR YOU TO TRAVEL TO A
PATIENT'S HOME? TIME _____ MILES _____

PLEASE NOTE ANY TRAVEL RESTRICTIONS OR OTHER CONSIDERATIONS _____
_____

TIME AVAILABILITY: PLEASE CHECK ALL TIME SLOTS IN WHICH YOU COULD
VOLUNTEER YOUR TIME.

Figure 17. Hospice Volunteer Application (Page 2)

	SUN	MON	TUES	WED	THURS	FRI	SAT
MORNING	___	___	___	___	_____	___	___
AFTERNOON	___	___	___	___	_____	___	___
EVENING	___	___	___	___	_____	___	___

What are your special skills/hobbies? _____
_____

What do you do for fun? _____
_____

WHY DO YOU WISH TO BE A HOSPICE VOLUNTEER? _____
_____
_____
_____
_____
_____

LANGUAGES SPOKEN FLUENTLY _____

Would you be willing to sign a contract outlining your responsibilities
as a Hospice volunteer? ___ YES   ___ NO

Can you make at least a one-year commitment to working as a Hospice
volunteer? ___ YES   ___ NO

If there is anything else you would like to mention, please feel free to
do so below. Thank you.

REFERENCES:
1. Name _____ Occupation _____
    Address _____ Phone (___)_____
             No./Street   City   Zip

2. Name _____ Occupation _____
    Address _____ Phone (___)_____
             No./Street   City   Zip

3. Name _____ Occupation _____
    Address _____ Phone (___)_____
             No./Street   City   Zip

                          _____
                          Signature

                          _____
                          Date

Figure 17. Hospice Volunteer Application (Page 3)

DATE: _____

TIME: _____

TELEPHONE INQUIRIES FOR HOSPICE SERVICES

NAME OF CALLER: _____
               Last   First   Middle

HOME ADDRESS: _____ ZIP _____ PHONE: (___)_____

BUSINESS ADDRESS: _____ PHONE: (___)_____

HOW DID YOU HEAR ABOUT OUR HOSPICE? _____

TYPE OF SERVICES REQUESTED: _____

_____

_____

PATIENT'S NAME: _____ AGE: ____ PHONE: (___)____

DIAGNOSIS: _____ LIFE EXPECTANCY: _____

PATIENT'S LOCATION: _____

REFERRAL: _____

_____

_____

COMMENTS:

_____

SIGNATURE: _____

TITLE: _____

Figure 18. Telephone Inquiries for Hospice Services

HOSPICE INTAKE SHEET

Date: _____ Time: _____ a.m. _____ p.m.

Interviewer: _____

PATIENT:

Name: _____ Sex _____

Address: _____

_____ Zip _____

Phone: (___)_____ SS #: _____

D.O.B.: _____ Age: _____ Marital Status: _____

Next of Kin:

Name: _____

Address: _____

Relationship: _____ Age: ____ Sex: _____

Phone: (___)_____

Primary Careperson (if different from above):

Name: _____ Age: ____ Sex: _____

Address: _____

Phone: (___)_____

REFERRAL:

How did you hear about Hospice? _____

_____

Name: _____

Professional Affiliation: _____

_____

Phone: (___)_____

Figure 19. Hospice Intake Sheet (Page 1)

HOSPICE INTAKE SHEET (continued)

MEDICAL:

Physician: _____

Address: _____

_____

Phone: (___) _____

DIAGNOSIS: _____

Date made: _____ Known by Patient _____ Family _____

Prognosis: _____ Known by Patient _____ Family _____

Most recent hospitalization date: _____

Name of Hospital: _____

Surgical History/other information _____

_____

Chemo: Active ____ Completed _____ Date _____ Refused _____

Radiation: Active ____ Completed _____ Date _____ Refused _____

Hormonal: _____

Current Treatments: _____

_____

INSURANCE CARRIER:

Primary   Secondary
_____   _____

Insured's Name   Insured's Name

Policy # _____Policy # _____

DIRECTIONS TO HOME: _____

_____

_____

OTHER: _____

_____

Figure 19. Hospice Intake Sheet (Page 2)

INDEX

ABOUT THE AUTHORS

The name of **Virginia F. Sendor,** MS, MPA, is synonymous with Hospice, a movement that believes dying is part of the life cycle and living with dignity is the right of every terminally ill human being. In 1985, she founded the Long Island Foundation for Hospice Care and Research, Inc., a nonprofit community-based organization committed to providing a certified program of comprehensive Hospice care to terminally ill patients and their families as an alternative to conventional curative care.

She was executive director of Life-Care Hospice, a fully certified Medicare/Medicaid agency that served all of Nassau County and western Suffolk County. She continues to serve on the Long-Term Care Task Force of the Nassau-Suffolk Health Systems Agency, Inc., and formerly also served on their Health Care Planning and Policy Committee and the Hospice Sub-Committee. She is on the Executive Board and is Hospice consultant to the Foundation of Thanatology and the American Institute for Life-Threatening Illness and Loss at Columbia Presbyterian Medical Center, as well as other groups. She is a member of the National Hospice Organization, New York State Hospice Association, Children's Hospice International, American Counseling Association, and the International Association for Near-Death Studies.

Ms. Sendor recently completed her MPA degree in health care administration and gerontology at Long Island University/C.W. Post Campus and was recognized by the New York State Legislature "for her long and sustained commitment to the preservation and enhancement of human dignity and her outstanding leadership in the Hospice movement."

Patrice M. O'Connor, RN, MA, CNA, has been an administrator in the Hospice/palliative care field for seventeen years. She is a Palliative Care Consultant, and was a consultant to the Palliative

Care Education Service at St. Luke's/Roosevelt Hospital Center in New York City. She was the Director of the St. Luke's Hospice/Palliative Care Program for twelve years—the first Hospice in a teaching hospital with a scattered-bed consultative team. Ms. O'Connor has lectured both nationally and internationally on Hospice and palliative care. She has also published on the subjects of spiritual care; administration and management of hospital-based Hospice/palliative care programs; music as a facilitator for coping; patients' last hours; humor as a part of living and dying; and dying in the hospital setting. She has done research and published in areas of attitudinal study of Hospice workers in providing spiritual care; effects of Medicare regulations on access to Hospice care; effects of inner-city palliative care service on inpatient utilization; an attitudinal study of health care workers concerning issues of dying/death; a study of a medical record audit of terminal care; and the effects of an educational intervention on staff's stress level and documentation.

Ms. O'Connor is a member of the International Work Group on Death, Dying and Bereavement, is founder and member of the Metropolitan Hospice and Palliative Care Association of New York City, and is on the United Hospital Fund Hospital Palliative Care Initiative Advisory Committee of New York City.